wellness
made simple

your guide to creating a sustainable,
holistic lifestyle by integrating
the 7 key factors of wellness

Laura Crooks

wellness made simple

A Laura Crooks Book
Copyright © 2014, **You Bloom Wellness**
All rights reserved.

Book Cover by Tracey Miller | www.TraceOfStyle.com
Publishing by Weston Lyon | www.WestonLyon.com
Edited by Lauren Cullumber

ISBN: 1500821675
EAN-13: 978-1500821678

This book contains opinions, ideas, experiences, and exercises - and is not intended as medical and/or health advice. Please consult a medical professional before adopting any of the suggestions in this book.

This book is dedicated to everyone
on a journey to wellness.

• • • •

Thanks to everyone who supports
me on my journey.

wellness made simple

table of contents

first things first 7

health vs. wellness 13

1 - integrated 17

2 - mindset 27

3 - time management 63

4 - stress management 69

5 - eating 89

6 - sleep 103

7 - exercise 115

8 - happiness 131

9 - motivation 139

10 - integrated again 147

your next step 151

about laura 153

first things first

why read this book

Most likely you've picked up this book because you're not satisfied with your current state of wellness, life-balance, overwhelm, energy, fitness level or happiness. This book is designed to help you with those areas of your life and help you actively participate in your journey of wellness.

Wellness Made Simple explains the process of creating a lifestyle of wellness. It follows my coaching process and presents a simple, holistic approach to making better decisions about your health and wellness. This book is an overview of the interrelated components of wellness: mindset, time management, stress management, eating, sleep, exercise, happiness, and motivation.

It is designed to be practical, encouraging and to spark action. In this book I present wellness as a holistic lifestyle with you as the decision maker. Wellness has many customizable versions and is about doing better and making progress for yourself, not you achieving the same goal as 50 other people.

In this book I am not telling you what to do; I don't believe there is a one-size-fits-all solution hiding out there. The ideas presented are not linear; you do not start here, do this and end up there. That may be frustrating for you if you're looking for THE answer.

Living well is a fluid process and there are many "right" ways to do it. *Wellness Made Simple* is a guidebook that encourages you to either start or continue on your journey of creating balance, happiness, and living well.

why I wrote this book

Through my years as a nurse and a coach I have watched people search for the "magic bullet" and the "quick fix" to health: the right way to eat, the right way to exercise, the best or fastest pill to help them achieve a desired result. While barreling along that highway they often miss their exit and start over and over on that same stretch of road. We can't undo years of poor decisions in a week.

The solution is not found in a quick fix but in a series of better decisions, or a lifestyle. Quick fixes are simply not a sustainable way to live. They tend to be harsh and drastic and focused on giving something up just until a desired result is achieved. A lifestyle, however, is an ongoing and gentle way of approaching each day as an opportunity to make better decisions. A lifestyle incorporates a variety of aspects of life.

This book is the foundation of my wellness coaching. No matter what people come to me wanting to achieve in their wellness or health, we always circle back to these core things: mindset, time management, sleep, stress management, happiness, eating and exercise.

I do not have all the answers but I can ask questions that help you find your answers. I do know there is no one right way to eat, live, sleep, exercise, or relax. Your journey to wellness will have some things in common with everyone else's journey but it will also look different. We might all enjoy "nice weather" but define the specifics differently.

There is no one best way for everyone to eat or exercise, nor is there a perfect way to reduce stress or a magic number of hours to sleep. We are all similar, yet unique. We are also living in real time, and what worked two years ago may not be working well now. Your wellness is unique to you at any given time in your life.

Most of us need to slow down, listen to our bodies and commit to a journey of wellness. It is an enjoyable journey, if you are the creator. Your wellness journey is not one that someone else can push or pull you along on. Others can support you, but you need to start the process. I truly believe we are all capable of making monumental changes, one small step at a time. It is not necessarily easy, but it really is simple.

Current research supports that your environment and your daily choices are supremely important in, and capable of, changing how your genetic destiny is expressed. This means how well you manage your stress, the food you choose to eat, your exercise and sleep can have equal, if not greater, influence on how well you feel and whether you develop disease than whether you carry a genetic trait for a disease. So even if a majority of your family developed type 2 diabetes it does not mean you have to. Your choices can affect that outcome.

Keep an open mind about trying new things, even things you think you won't like: new foods, new thought patterns, new ways of exercising, a new sleep schedule, new ways of relaxing. If you are reading this book because what you are currently doing is isn't working, what have you got to lose?

I want this book to give you hope and inspiration for making better choices and taking the steering wheel of your wellness. I wrote it because there is so much we each can do to help ourselves but we get overwhelmed with the options or don't know where to start. I tried to make it simple, because there is enough confusion and overwhelm out there. This book can give you clarity or be your catalyst for change. The topics are circular - they all affect each other, because a lifestyle of wellness is not linear. It is an upward spiraling process.

before we begin:

health versus wellness

While I sometimes use the terms wellness and health interchangeably, I can make a distinction between the two. Wellness, to me, is a broader, more encompassing and more holistic term involving your body, mind, and spirit while health implies an absence of disease and a more medical assessment of the parts or systems of the body.

When we work on our health we compartmentalize our body systems and tend to start with the system or part that seems the most broken (and we often let things get pretty broken before intervening). We work to improve that one aspect and consider it done when we are told there is no more disease, we have halted the disease progression, or we have reached our expected improvement. We stop working on it and either coast until it flares up and breaks again or shift our attention to the next ailing body part. Health is fairly black and white, usually centered on defining what is not functioning well or being told there is no disease.

For example, even though you have not been feeling well you put off (maybe for years) seeing your doctor, and therefore, do not receive the diagnosis of high blood pressure (or cancer, or diabetes…). Does not having the diagnosis make you healthy? Were you healthy the hour before getting your diagnosis and only became unhealthy once diagnosed? Once you get the diagnosis or disease label, does it change the way you think about your wellness and health? It often does because being healthy means not getting a diagnosis and not failing the health "test." We often let our health or diagnosis define us.

Wellness focuses more on all the things that are going well and areas in which you are making positive improvements. Wellness is a sense of living to your potential and functioning optimally. You can have a diagnosis, even a terminal illness, and live with a sense of wellness because being well is a process and not a definition.

Wellness has an internal approach. It involves listening to our bodies and promoting healing. Health has an external approach; we look outside of ourselves for treatment or a cure. The two are closely related and both have value.

I see wellness as a journey with you in the driver's seat and health more as a specific destination that you either arrive at or not. Health is choreographed by someone else and is centered on finding and fixing what is broken. Someone proclaims you to have (or not have) good health while your ongoing wellness lifestyle is created and coordinated by you. Wellness is a sustainable lifestyle consisting of a series of choices and decisions made entirely by you. Wellness emphasizes the positives.

Creating wellness is a sustainable way to live. It's not a crash course you hope to achieve by an unrealistic date, as in, "I need to lose 20 pounds by my class reunion in two weeks" or "I need to get my blood sugar numbers looking good by next week's lab work." Rome wasn't built in a day and you aren't going to change your beliefs and lifestyle in a day, either. But you can make new choices each day. So shift your mindset into enjoying the journey!

1

integrated

Wellness is about the way you move through the world; the way you live, think and act. It is not something you do occasionally or by scattering a few "healthier" activities or foods into your life. It is how you are with yourself, with others, and with the environment in general. It begins with your mindset and extends out to more visible behaviors.

We are much more than just a collection of body parts; we are whole, complete beings. Our body, mind and spirit function together as one to make us uniquely well. The premise of my belief about wellness is that our mindset, stress, sleep, happiness, eating, exercise and time management all affect each other and are in constant interaction. The underlying factor determining what we see ourselves capable of accomplishing is our mindset. How much we accomplish is affected by our time management. And motivation is what keeps the process going. So these are the chapters in *Wellness Made Simple*: mindset, time management, stress management, eating, sleep, exercise, happiness, and motivation.

The components of wellness all affect each other; they can create an upward spiral or a downward spiral. We do ourselves a disservice when we don't see ourselves as an integrated whole and don't appreciate the ease with which one part affects another.

We tend to separate different aspects of our wellness and associate each with a particular outcome: "I need to sleep more so I have more energy," "I need to eat less so I lose weight," "I need to exercise to manage my stress." These ideas are all valid, but incomplete. Losing weight is about more than reducing calories, feeling energetic is about more than getting enough sleep. Your food choices, stress, happiness, and activity level also affect your energy levels. Your sleep, stress, happiness and exercise affect your weight along with what you eat.

The way we nourish and rest our bodies affects how our bodies function. When and what we eat affects our sleep, stress, mood and energy level. Our stress affects our food choices, our mood and our sleep. Our exercise can affect our sleep, stress, energy, mood and weight. If we manage our time poorly we will undoubtedly say we don't have enough time to get enough sleep, cook healthy meals, manage our stress, do the activities we love, or exercise. As we get more frustrated with our perceived lack of time, and wellness seems farther and farther out of reach, our happiness plummets and our whole thought process changes.

Our friends and hobbies influence the way we eat and manage stress. Do you meet your friends for a movie, an all-afternoon house painting party, or time spent gardening together? Our job affects how and when we move. An ironworker moves differently than a trim carpenter, an ICU nurse moves differently than a school nurse, and a college professor moves differently than a kindergarten teacher. Our social supports and relationships affect our mood and what we eat. Do your friends cheer you up with wings and margaritas or a night out dancing? Does your office celebrate with donuts or a softball game?

When we sleep appropriately, we reset our appetite hormones. Sleep also helps manage stress; without a good night's sleep we may feel impatient, cranky, and intolerant of unexpected events. The effects of chronic stress from running late, rude people, traffic jams, and misplaced items accumulate and can trigger mindless munching, emotional eating, and rushed and less than nutritious food choices. Poor food choices contribute to feeling slug-

gish, which make us less inclined to exercise or cook nutritious foods. Stress, fatigue, and low energy levels affect
our mood, making us feel irritable which makes us less
happy. Our fatalistic, negative thinking and failed weight
loss attempts eventually persuade us that we are incapa-
ble of achieving or maintaining weight loss.

Eating, exercising, sleep and stress management all affect our willpower or self-control. When we are hungry,
tired and drained from chronic stress we feel our willpower vanish. Then we start the downward slide of letting
one bad decision create another until we are berating ourselves and feeling like we can do no better.

In the concept of wellness, as opposed to health, we have
an inner locus of control. Our bodies have a complete and
innate wisdom and it behooves us to listen. In the concept
of health, someone else proclaims us to be whole and
healthy (free of disease) and because we are listening to
someone else we often stop listening to our body. We
were born knowing instinctively how to get our needs met
but gradually stopped listening to our inner wisdom and
overrode our instincts.

The internal approach is to listen to your body. You knew how to do this as a baby; you slept when tired, relaxed, laughed and moved daily, and ate when you were hungry. In early childhood we learned to override our instincts and ate when we weren't hungry, stayed up too late fighting sleep, and gradually had less and less play, movement and relaxation in our day.

So, a lot of your wellness journey is not learning something new but re-learning old skills. You don't have to start the process of wellness from scratch but you do need to unlearn your current habits. You need to quiet your current mindset and behaviors so you can hear your inner wisdom.

When you change your mindset, the way you think about yourself, your weight, lifestyle and possibilities in general, your behaviors change to align with your new thinking patterns. It is not a quick fix, but a permanent, sustainable new lifestyle.

body - mind - spirit

We are whole, integrated beings complete with a body, mind, and spirit that each factor into our wellness. Your body needs good food, exercise and rest to perform at its best. Your mind needs both stimulation and relaxation. Nourishing your spirit means living with a sense of purpose and connectedness.

You are a three-legged stool, with one leg each for body, mind, and spirit. When one leg is too short or too long, you feel stressed, restless, or unwell. You feel well when your body, mind, and spirit are in harmony.

These integrated parts of wellness all affect each other:

- mindset
- sleep
- stress management
- eating
- exercise
- happiness
- time management
- and your motivation affects your perseverance in making sustainable lifestyle changes.

Each leg of the stool needs a different amount of attention to achieve a balanced length. We are naturally better at caring for one leg of our stool, and which leg that is can change over the years. The amount of attention each needs changes over time as our skills and needs change. We need to find the balance of how much attention to give our dominant and non-dominant legs. Some people are naturally resilient, happy and relaxed. While their "mind leg" might be naturally strong they may need to pay careful attention to how they care for their physical body. To someone else balancing their weight or getting enough exercise might come easily but they need to consciously nurture their sense of connectedness and purpose. Each leg of your stool does need some attention, but each leg does not need the same amount.

Wellness is creating the optimal balance between body, mind, and spirit. When one leg is just a little shorter or longer than the others we may feel a little dissatisfied or a little less well than usual. When our "legs" are very uneven we might feel like a wreck and very unwell. We should periodically check in with what parts of our lives are running smoothly and to what parts we could devote more time and attention.

Often we hit a point when we realize that the things that have worked well in the past either no longer work well or that things have gotten way off track with regard to paying attention to our wellness. It may take something as drastic as a health wake up call for us to take back the steering wheel and redesign our wellness. Sometimes just a general feeling of not being at our peak can even trigger it. Working to rebalance our body, mind and spirit can put us back on track to managing our wellness.

Our weight can be a perfect example of various systems affecting each other. Our stress level affects our sleep and our sleep affects our stress. You have probably felt grumpy, less patient and more overwhelmed after a night or two short on sleep. Without enough sleep, our appetite hormones do not reset properly, leaving us craving sweet and fatty foods, feeling hungrier than usual and less likely to feel full or satisfied after eating. We make poor food choices because we are tired and stressed; we are then less inclined to plan and prepare a healthy meal. We seek convenient comfort foods, but less healthy foods can further sap our energy, making us more fatigued and less likely to exercise. This then leads us to sit on the couch, not exercising and eating even more junk food.

This becomes a cycle when the stress of watching ourselves gain weight and feeling less energetic causes our self-talk to become more negative. As we berate ourselves and feel like we can do nothing right we convince ourselves we might as well keep eating and we then proceed to either eat even more or we decide to punish ourselves and skip a few meals. But by starving ourselves

and not eating good food at regular intervals (this includes skipping breakfast or lunch to push through our
busy day) we become overly hungry by late afternoon.
We then eat readily-available junk food and realize that
we overate, as we sag once again onto the couch feeling
stuffed before slumping into a subsequent plunge in blood
sugar.

This unhealthy lifestyle loop can be reversed by making
small positive changes anywhere along the cycle. We
could start by getting more sleep and directly improve our
mood, appetite, energy levels, and patience so we are
more likely to cook, exercise, and stay calm. Or we could
start by adding some relaxation exercises, which might
help us sleep better and do less stress eating. Exercise
can be both a stress reliever and sleep enhancer. Exercise can shift our mindset to a more positive state where
we are more inclined to make healthier lifestyle choices
overall. It can burn fat and tone muscles, giving added
motivation to clean up our eating or take care of our bodies in other ways. How we manage our time dictates how
we spend each minute and whether we make time for
wellness.

Your mindset is involved because the thoughts you think affect your stress level, your food choices, your propensity to exercise and your sleep. When you think angry or fearful thoughts your body responds with stress, more muscle tension, and an increased heart rate. Emotional eating can spike and your stress hormones send you in search of sugary, fatty pick-me-ups. When you think peaceful, loving thoughts, your mind opens, your heart rate and breathing slow, and your stress response changes. You are more likely to take care of yourself when you have positive thoughts.

You, as a 3-legged stool:

Imagine yourself as a 3-legged stool with a body, mind, and spirit leg. Each leg must be a similar length to the other legs so that you feel balanced and well.

2

mindset

Your thoughts and beliefs shape your wellness. Your mindset affects your approach to taking care of yourself and becomes the base on which your future actions rest. How you perceive your capabilities and how you think about your role in your wellness directly impact your sleep, stress, eating, exercise and happiness.

knowing versus doing

There is a huge difference between knowing something and doing it. Knowing it is in your head, doing it is in your actions. You can know how to change a tire but not do it, you can know how to cook vegetables but not do it. You can also know that you would be better off if you exercised and got enough sleep. But knowing these things and doing them are different skill sets. It can be difficult to apply your knowledge. You may need to unlearn some habits as you create new ones. Some things we know seem so simple but are difficult to implement.

27

Sometimes we need to start the process by better under-standing what and why we want to change. Other times we know full well what we want to do. We often need to break the process into smaller steps, get support for mak-ing the changes, and just start *doing.*

Knowing what to do does not guarantee you will do it. Ac-knowledge the difference between the two and put sup-ports, accountability and reminders into the "doing" part of the process.

mind-body link

Your mind and body are intricately intertwined and do af-fect each other. You can alter your physiology just by changing your thoughts. When you think of something that scares or angers you, you can feel your heart rate climb and your muscles tense. You can actually put your-self in a bad mood just by thinking about negative things. You can also feel your heart rate and breathing settle down by thinking of happy, loving, or calming thoughts. Picturing yourself in a soothing place surrounded by peo-ple who love you can change your physiology for the bet-ter.

thoughts drive behaviors

Your thoughts drive your beliefs and emotions, which drive your behaviors. If you see the glass as half empty you will find "evidence" of that everywhere. If you are in a bad mood or see yourself as having little or no control in a situation your actions will reflect that. If you think the world is full of mean, scheming people you will always notice those people. In finding evidence to support your beliefs you may not see the kind, genuine and generous people.

If you think that people won't like you, you'll be less likely to introduce yourself to others or meet new people. Because you believe you are not someone others will find interesting, you will not see opportunities to meet others or put yourself in social situations. But if you believe that others will find you interesting you will be more likely to go places where you can meet people.

If you believe you are less than capable, you will not try as hard or as often. And you will be less likely to see ways to improve your capabilities.

If you believe that your health is all a matter of genes and destiny you probably think that nothing you do will matter in the long run, so why bother changing your lifestyle. If, on the other hand, you do feel your actions make a difference, you will be more likely to take care of yourself and make proactive choices. How we think about our health and wellness influences the decisions we make and the actions we take.

Let your attitude drive your behaviors. What is your attitude about your health and wellness and your role in them? If you believe you are pre-programmed to develop certain diseases by a particular age, because that is what happened to Mom and Uncle Bob, then you will be less likely to take an active and preventative approach to your health. If you believe you have diabetes because "it is in my genes" then you will be less likely to make better lifestyle choices and accept your participation in how the disease plays out.

change

Change begins with awareness and relies on action. First, taking action in aligning your mindset with your desired outcomes and second, taking action or changing your behaviors. We are capable of change thanks to neuroplasticity. Our brains are capable of making new connections between neurons and restructuring based on our thoughts and actions. We used to think that once we reached adulthood our brains were wired in a fixed way. Luckily, they are not. We are all capable of change.

Your mindset, or basic beliefs, about living well are what change your actions from behaviors that culminate in a one-time goal to creating and living a journey of wellness; it is a process. You don't just achieve wellness or health once and say it's done. You create wellness over and over, day after day, decision after decision. It becomes an ongoing, perpetual way of thinking and living.

A dieter might make drastic choices to lose weight but when they reach their target weight they stop dieting, revert to their original habits and often gain weight. Someone who maintains weight loss makes sustainable choices over and over and has created a new lifestyle to support their new weight.

Someone who believes that relaxation and managing stress are important to their wellness will restructure their day to make time for relaxation and look for ways to alter stressful situations.

There are many theories on change. Some promote making changes in many areas simultaneously and as you have small successes you create a bigger upward spiral of success. Another approach is to make one change at a time and master that before moving to the next. By focusing on just one thing at a time you will avoid overwhelm and feel mastery. Some people seem to do better with one approach than another, and the same goes for certain areas of change. For most people making lifestyle changes, I suggest making small changes in several areas simultaneously. Since the components of wellness are interrelated and affect one another, making small dents in several aspects can speed up the feeling of success in creating a better lifestyle.

> *"Change begins with awareness and relies on action."*
>
> Laura Crooks

stages of change

There are different degrees of willingness to change and those stages can vary by topic and time. You may not be at all ready or willing to make changes in the way you eat, but you are ready to enhance your sleep routine and have been thinking about reducing your stress but are unsure where to start. The stages of change range from absolutely not wanting to change at all, to considering it, to feeling ready, to having started making changes but needing support to continue, to having successfully made and maintained the changes for some time. You won't be successful in forcing yourself to make changes in areas where you are not ready. As you read each chapter, decide how willing you are to make a change within each topic.

Beginning to take action does not mean jumping to the final goal. In starting to address your sleep you may need to track how long you sleep each night and how long it takes you to get ready to go to bed. If you want to add more fiber to your diet you may need to research foods high in fiber then find recipes for them. Research and planning comes before shopping, which comes before actually eating the new food. When you do start eating higher fiber foods you may start with only one meal a week, gradually increasing to one meal a day.

maintaining change

Maintaining an achievement takes a different mindset and different set of actions than initially achieving it. You can't maintain changes unless your thoughts and beliefs support the changes. That is why your mindset is so crucial to improving your wellness. The way you think about your wellness and health drives your behaviors.

Consider weight loss. You employ certain behaviors to lose the weight but even after you achieve your desired weight, the process is not over. You continue the maintenance behaviors...forever if that is how long you want to stay at your desired weight. Similarly, beginning an exercise program looks very different from maintaining one. As a beginner you may exercise for a much shorter period of time, or you may repeat the same motion over and over until you are comfortable with it. You may use lighter weights or complete an easier course than someone more experienced. As you begin, you need to consciously think about doing it. Once you have achieved success with it and it has become a habit, you just do it. You can enjoy the movement without having to think about each step. Remember learning to drive? It initially took a lot of concentration to distinguish the gas pedal from the brake, whether the left turn signal was moving the lever up or down, and how to gauge when to start braking. After a while you just drove without consciously thinking about each step in the process.

The maintenance behaviors need to be sustainable, something you can live with every day; they need to become your new way of living. A lifestyle incorporates behaviors, whereas a temporary fix applies a new layer of behaviors over the existing ones, and you peel off that temporary layer as soon as your goals are met. Maintaining and achieving behaviors may overlap.

Friends tend to offer support and acknowledgement while we are achieving, but rarely acknowledge our efforts at maintaining, despite our ongoing work and attention. Ask anyone who has lost weight and kept it off or quit smoking. People offer praise and support during the initial phase, but how often does anyone let them know they are doing a great job at maintaining their new healthier lifestyle three years out? It is human nature to notice the initial change then move on. Just keep in mind that you will need to be your biggest supporter of maintenance efforts.

> *"Achieving and maintaining change are two different skill sets."*
>
> Laura Crooks

conscious and subconscious thoughts

We have conscious thoughts, those that we are aware of, and subconscious thoughts, those that we are not aware of. Our brain tries to validate what we are thinking by letting us "see" things that support our beliefs, even those in our subconscious.

You see more of what you pay attention to. If you are feeling hurt or angry you naturally see things around you to support that feeling. When you think positive and grateful thoughts you naturally see more things to affirm those beliefs. We don't want to be wrong, so we find supporting evidence for whatever we are thinking.

When you are planning a vacation, ads or pictures of places similar to those you plan to visit catch your eye more than ads for baby diapers. But if you are pregnant you notice the baby diaper ads and all the other pregnant women around you. That is because babies are on your mind and your brain searches for more of what you are thinking about.

We are often not even aware of our thoughts. They are always with us and we are used to them; they are what we carry in our head each day. We have had them for so long and they are the only lens we are accustomed to looking through. We take our conscious thoughts for granted and are not even aware of our subconscious thoughts. Our subconscious thoughts may include beliefs and habits we acquired as children. They could include values and beliefs about money, religion, education, food, friends, appearance, or anything. Recognizing our thoughts and beliefs can be tough, but we need to notice our thoughts to be able to change them and then change our outcomes.

If you believe you are destined to be overweight because your parents were overweight your behaviors around managing your weight will be very different from someone who believes they have some control and that their choices affect their weight. This may or may not be something you are conscious of.

If you believe you "need" your stress to help you perform and meet deadlines you will take a different approach to managing your stress than someone who thinks their abundance of stress may be negatively impacting their life and health.

If you know you do not sleep much but believe there are simply not enough hours in the day and you must sacrifice sleep to get everything else done you will probably not change the amount you sleep. If, however, you think there might be a way to streamline or forego something from your day, you are more likely to get more sleep.

Think about the areas in which you want to see positive improvements. What are your underlying beliefs about your role in those areas? Are your thoughts on each issue predominantly positive and hopeful? Do you see yourself as capable of gathering the resources to make the desired change? Or do you see your destiny as being written in stone or insurmountable? Long-term success comes when our beliefs and actions are aligned.

Do you believe you can successfully manage your stress, maintain your ideal weight, or improve your wellness?

positive or negative thoughts

It is estimated that we think about 60,000 thoughts a day and that about 70% or our thoughts are negative. Even positive, upbeat people have a predominance of negative self-talk, the commentary in our head.

The ticker tape of chatter and self-talk in our head is often about what went wrong, what might go wrong, how we don't measure up, deficits, defects, fear, anger and insecurity. Pessimistic, critical, complaining, whining, blaming, accusing, jealous, resentful, self-pitying, inferior and belittling thoughts are also all negative. We are essentially continuously beating ourselves up.

If we all tend to find or create more of what is in our minds, what are we creating with all these negative thoughts? Begin to notice your thoughts. Notice whether your thoughts are supportive and uplifting or degrading and negative. After becoming aware of your thoughts, begin replacing negative thoughts with positive or at least neutral thoughts. "I'm not good enough to get that job" becomes "I can give that job a shot" or "I can do that," or even, "What can I do to feel more qualified?" "I'm such a klutz" becomes "I dropped the chips and I will clean them up." "I'm such a loser because I skipped spinning class again" can be "I missed spinning class, where can I fit in a run?"

Simply replacing negative thoughts with positive thoughts can leave you feeling better now but not necessarily change the underlying beliefs. But by repeating new actions you can change your beliefs. Start by noticing your thoughts, then changing them to something more positive, then follow that with forward-moving actions. After a while you can believe that you truly are capable.

sense of control

Something as subtle as how you word your thoughts can affect you. Consider the following two sentences (say them out loud to feel the difference): "I should do laundry today" versus "I could do laundry today." Generally thoughts with "should" in them feel like an oppressive burden placed upon you. Thoughts with "could" imply we have a choice and feel a bit lighter. We like to feel we have some control in a situation and "could" lets us feel that power to choose. Choosing to do something has internal origins.

A perceived sense of control puts us in the driver's seat. We often have greater follow through when we feel we chose to do something. A sense of power contributes to a sense of hope, which changes the playing field. The combination of hope and control makes us much more likely to do something.

Compare the feeling of the words "must" or "have to" with the word "choose." "I have to walk after dinner" feels different than "I choose to walk after dinner." "I must finish all of these wings" feels different from "I choose to finish all of the wings." "Must" makes it a foregone conclusion that those wings will be eaten while "choose to" causes us to step back and ask, "What did I say?" Simply rewording your thoughts so that you have a choice can improve your success of actually following through.

"The fries came with the entrée, so I have to eat them," has an external source of control. You are eating the fries because you choose to frame the situation as one where it was out of your control. "I choose to have fries with lunch," means you have total ownership over that behavior and you will probably think twice about doing it.

Change is based on a series of choices. We often erode or underestimate our power of choice by saying things like, "I didn't have a choice," "What choice did I have?" "Things happen," "I'm unlucky," or "It was just bound to be this way." We have more choices than we realize and we need to start seeing our behaviors as choices.

Sometimes your only choice is to choose how you respond to or think about a situation. You always have the choice of how to think about something. Things do happen that are beyond your control, such as when a water main breaks and you have no water for a day. You do not control the water, but you do control how you think about and respond to the situation.

hope

Hope is an important part of the mindset of wellness. Hope drives healing and lets us make better choices. Hope is tied to our sense of control. When we feel hopeless and that we have no power in a situation we take on a defeatist attitude and do not make the same proactive choices. Hope is linked to optimism, which is linked to positive thinking. So practicing gratitude, which can boost your positive thinking, can make you more hopeful. Seeing your choices in each setting gives you a sense of control and power; you can control whether you make better choices.

do you believe

Do you believe you can make positive changes and improve your health or wellness? The key to being able to do something is believing that you can. You not only need to be ready, willing and able, but you need the confidence to begin. We all have things we are considering doing sometime in the future. The fact that we aren't doing it yet means something is not ready for us to proceed with the idea. Sometimes we aren't able because we don't have the resources (information, time, money, or support) and sometimes we just aren't willing (we lack the motivation or desire) and sometimes we just aren't ready (we lack the confidence or it is just not realistic now).

Making changes, even positive ones, can be challenging and takes ongoing work. Before you start you need to be ready, willing and able to change; you need the resources, the incentive or motivation and the capability.

confidence

Feeling confident is a combination of how you view yourself and your skills in relation to the circumstances. Some
people are naturally more confident than others, and no
one feels 100% confident in all situations. Our perspective and whether we take action or not influence our confidence. Confidence grows as we successfully take action.
So if you never try something your confidence in it will
never grow.

Sometimes having the confidence to begin is tied to how
we clarify our goal and identify the next step. Desired outcomes that are too big and hazy do not inspire confidence; they scare or overwhelm us. When the next step
is unclear we feel less certain. One technique to over-
coming this is to see the big goal, then shrink it down to a
size you can work with this week. Are you aiming to lose
50 pounds, or 1 pound and repeating it 49 times? Are you
planning to write a book or one paragraph, which then
leads to another? Are you focusing on eating seven cups
of fruits and vegetables a day or one cup of vegetables
with today's dinner?

It takes courage to take each small action step. And with
each step taken your confidence grows. The key to build-

ing confidence is taking action, continually taking small steps. With each accomplishment you become more self-assured.

If you don't think you can, you might never try. Gradually change your thinking then add action to back it up.

strengths

Start noticing your strengths. We all have gifts. What do you do well? What would your friends describe as your talents? Are you curious and fun loving? Are you tenacious and follow tasks through to completion? Are you caring and empathetic? Are you logical or whimsical? Are you rational and calm in a crisis? Are you the visionary, the leader, or the worker bee? Recognizing your strengths as strengths lets you draw on a wide range of skills and attributes moving forward.

Traits that you view as a weakness or even a flaw probably have a flip side and can be viewed as a strength in other settings. Being loud, pushy and stubborn may be just what is needed in a crisis but not necessarily the best response in a sensitive negotiation. Being accommodating, agreeable and nurturing may be called for when helping a friend through trying times, but is not helpful in an evacuation.

Notice what you do well and apply it to your advantage. If you recognize your ability to make a to-do list and follow it as a strength you can consciously apply that technique to adding in healthier behaviors; write your healthy behaviors as a to-do list. If you can recognize yourself as a compassionate and caring friend, turn that strength toward yourself and be gentle with yourself as you move forward making lifestyle changes.

Recognizing your strengths does not mean you sit around egotistically beating your chest, nurturing a massive ego. It means having a realistic and positive view of your skills and attributes. As you acknowledge your strengths and you will begin to see more benefits of them and more situations that capitalize on them.

alternate truths

A dime has two very different sides. Neither side is better or more right than the other.

There is always more than one way to view a situation. Learning to see an alternate truth is important in opening your mindset. There is more than one right way to make potato salad, paint a picture or manage your stress. Sometimes we defeat our own efforts simply by the way we wrap meaning into something.

You set out to lose 75 pounds and lose 70. Is that success or failure? Wasn't there success in those 70 pounds?

You always have at least two donuts at work on Fridays. You promised yourself you wouldn't have any this week but you ate half a donut. Is that good or bad, improvement or defeat?

Is following a schedule liberating or confining? It could be either: by following a schedule you can free up time for fun or you can crowd fun out.

Is a schedule set in stone or a guideline?

Is a to-do list a mandatory activity sheet or a list of suggestions?

You planned to join a gym last weekend, researched a few, and even visited some but never actually bought the membership because a friend needed help when their dog ran away. Is what you did good or bad? You did the prep work for joining a gym and you also helped a friend do something that couldn't wait.

You want to cook dinners at home more often but don't know what to make, so you spend an afternoon researching recipes, planning meals and making a shopping list. Do you see that afternoon as time well spent or as time not spent cleaning the garage, which was on the to-do list?

Get your mind in order:

- notice and then change your negative thoughts.
- know your personal strengths and work with them.
- see the alternate truths.
- plan ahead.
- practice self-compassion.
- measure progress.

Is eating healthy food, but way too much of it a good thing or a bad thing? Could it be an event that has both some good and some bad?

There are no right answers. There are only options on how you view each.

Is the glass half full, half empty, or both? We tend to auto-matically jump to one conclusion or the other. Just be aware that a situation can contain good things and still leave room for improvement.

progress, not perfection

As you move forward you should be looking for signs of progress. Drop the expectation that things will or even should be perfect. Mistakes will be made, side journeys and detours will be taken. Allow yourself to see the vari-ous shades of gray between the black and white end-points. Categorizing everything as white or black, good or bad, right or wrong, doesn't let you give yourself credit for the beneficial actions you did take.

Let's say you are trying to meditate daily for 10 minutes and this past week you meditated for five days. Is that a success or failure? You did not do it all seven days, but you did do it five times, which is more than you used to do. Let's say you did not manage to meditate at all last week but you figured out that you need to set aside a specific time in the morning so you can be successful. While you did not succeed in meditating you did learn something helpful about the process. You discovered information that can propel you forward.

With a black and white mindset you would only see the failure. With a non-supportive mindset you will berate yourself for what you did not achieve. With a supportive and open mindset you can appreciate the new information, give yourself credit where credit is due and move on without rehashing the failure and building the negatives in your mind.

The classic example of progress, not perfection, is a baby learning to walk. It is expected that there will be falls and that the first few attempts will not be steady or even successful. But the baby keeps trying, we keep cheering him on and eventually the baby can walk. Each individual step then adds up to miles. Hiking the Appalachian Trail starts with the first step, which is followed by the second step. After lots of steps you may complete the trail but it would not have been possible without each of the individual small steps.

No one is holding you to an expectation of perfection. Why do you expect perfection of yourself?

preventing slip ups

While creating new habits it can be useful to eliminate some of the cracks you can fall into. Minimize your daily variability and eliminate as many decisions as you can. When we have choices to make we often stop, lose our forward momentum and open the door to falling off the wagon.

Whatever it is you are working on try doing it the same way every day for a week. Eat the same breakfast, pack the same lunch, exercise at the same time, go to sleep and wake up at the same time, do the same relaxation exercise in the same place.

When things look the same every day you don't have to stop and wonder whether you should treat yourself to fries today, whether you will exercise later if you hit the snooze button, whether you could watch one more episode, or whether you should take five minutes to file today's papers. You can decide to eat only one square of dark chocolate right after dinner; now you don't need to wonder about whether you should have dessert with lunch or what to have for dessert after dinner. If you commit to drinking one glass of water before your first cup of coffee, then it's pretty clear what to do, you don't need to think about it. You make the decision to do the new habit when you are well fed, rested and feeling good and strong. Then you don't need to think about that again.

Commit to this for one week, then renew the commitment if it helped. Continue renewing the commitment until you have created a habit. I don't recommend living in a black and white world, but minimizing variability initially can really help establish the habit of doing a particular behavior.

slip-ups

Inevitably, slip-ups will happen. Your next decision is: how will you respond? Controlling your thoughts is something you can and should do. And you can pre-decide your response.

So you just missed your planned exercise opportunity - there was a traffic jam coming home and the commute took three times as long as expected. What do you tell yourself? "I ruined this week's exercise record so I'll start Monday (or next month, or January 1…)," "I don't have time to do a full workout but I can do five minutes now," or "I will make up for it tomorrow," or "Great, because I didn't want to exercise anyway!" Today's "slip-up" does not have to dictate tomorrow's action. You can restart right now. Shrink your starting time to each hour or each minute. Eating one piece of cake does not have to mean you must eat the whole cake or eat cake every day this week. As soon as you notice the behavior, ask yourself if that is what you want to continue doing. Would continuing that behavior move you toward your goal?

self-compassion

We tend to be harder on ourselves than we are on our friends. I ask that you treat yourself with the same kindness you would offer a friend. You can still drive yourself as hard as you would like, but if things do not turn out "perfectly" use some self-compassion and acknowledge what went well. And then plan for tomorrow.

Practicing self-compassion is not being self-indulgent and it is not letting yourself "get away" with anything. If a friend did not get a job they interviewed for, what would you tell them? And what would you tell yourself if it was you who did not get the job? The messages should be similar. Self-compassion actually helps you become more empathetic and have more patience.

forgiveness

The purpose of forgiving, or accepting, is to lessen the hold that past hurts have on your current thoughts and actions. In forgiving yourself and others, you acknowledge or accept that things have happened. You are not agreeing with the behaviors or outcomes, you are not saying they were acceptable or all right. You simply acknowledge they occurred. Remove the judgment from the action and stop blaming yourself, or others.

Harboring resentment, anger, guilt and grudges prevents you from moving forward; acknowledge they occurred and let them go. Allow yourself to accept that what happened, happened. You can neither control the past nor change it but you can accept it and move forward. Today's behaviors do not have to be rooted in your past; you have the strength to move beyond those behaviors.

Begin by identifying all of the people you need to forgive (including yourself).

What exactly are you forgiving each person for? Allow yourself time to sit with any emotions that surface. You can now make decisions from the mind of the new you, allowing your behaviors to be linked to your future, not your past.

actions and outcomes

As you make healthy lifestyle changes, keep in mind the distinction between actions and outcomes. You may take the action of being in bed ready to sleep by 10 PM each night but still find yourself having trouble achieving the outcome of being asleep by 10:15. You may be eating smaller portions but not losing the weight you wanted to lose. Maybe the desired outcome needs more action steps before it can happen. Just because you do not get the desired outcome does not mean the action was wrong. Give yourself credit for doing the action and think about what else might need to be added in to achieve the outcome.

planning ahead

Planning ahead is one of the most important skills in the wellness journey. Just like you would not throw random ingredients together and hope you end up with a delicious cake, you don't make random actions hoping something will come together and give you a specific desired result. Before a vacation you need to know where you are going so you know what type of items to bring and how long you will be there so you know how much to pack. You need to make arrangements for your pets, plants and what food you can leave in the fridge. Could you go on a trip without doing any of this? Of course. But you will probably have an easier and more enjoyable time away if you spend some time pre-planning.

It's the same with your journey to better wellness. Get in the habit of planning ahead: what is on your calendar for the next three days, when can you exercise and grocery shop, what meals will you prepare, what ingredients do you need? Is there anything really stress inducing coming up and how can you best prepare for the stress, is there a meeting during lunch that you should plan to eat either before or after? Make time regularly to gather your re-sources whether they are food, gym clothes, a way to un-wind at night, or recipes. Without good planning you may end your workday so hungry that the vending machine looks like a viable dinner option or find it is time for bed and you haven't exercised or done a relaxation exercise. A little time spent pre-planning saves time down the road and can prevent some less than ideal decisions.

plan B

Plan B is the back-up plan you make as you are planning ahead. Think about when and why "it" might not happen and make a contingency plan. What if your 11 AM meeting runs long and you miss lunch? What if you sleep through your alarm and don't have time to cook breakfast? What if your mom and aunt encourage you to eat desserts at the party?

We make better decisions when we are not in the heat of the moment, hungry, frustrated, or tired. Make an alternate plan for when your original plan falls through. If you know traffic on a certain road is terrible at 6 PM, you learn a different route, you create alternate options, or you change your timing. Do the same with your wellness.

reminders

Reminders are not only OK to use, they are necessary! You are creating new habits. This is hard work and takes time. You also need to remember what you are working on. It will be all too easy to start your day in your usual fashion and forget all about taking a moment to think of things for which you are grateful, especially when you are rushed or stressed. So accept that using reminders is a helpful tool, not a reflection of your inability to make changes. Use visual and/or auditory reminders until the new behavior becomes second nature - a new habit. Put notes where you need to see them (mirror, car seat or front door), set a phone alarm, put the jeans you want to fit into again front and center in your closet, or leave an item in an unusual place to remind you to do your new "something." Change your reminders every few days so you do not become accustomed to them; use a different color of paper for your note, put the note in a different spot.

Linking a new behavior to an established habit can make it easier to remember: put your toothbrush on your gratitude journal, put your vitamins in your coffee mug. You don't have to think twice about brushing your teeth or having a morning cup of coffee, so use those habits to remind you of your new habits-in-training.

We think it is silly to need reminders about something we want to do. It isn't silly. Create and use reminders until the behavior becomes a habit.

carrot or stick

What motivates you to make healthy lifestyle changes, gaining a reward (the carrot) or avoiding a consequence (the stick)? Are you more motivated by moving toward pleasure or away from pain? Are you gaining strength, energy, and a fit body or avoiding diabetes, high blood pressure and sluggish energy? In making lifestyle changes you can focus on what you are giving up (chips, channel surfing, late nights) or you can focus on what you will gain (an appreciation for real food, more effective ways of relaxing, feeling refreshed and rested).

Are you giving up a TV show or gaining an hour of sleep? Which motivates you more, achieving the goal (being fit enough to enjoy an active vacation, living to play with your grandchildren without complications from diabetes) or avoiding the consequence (obesity and a sedentary "watching from the sidelines" lifestyle, high blood pressure medicine, kidney failure and toe amputations)?

If you only focus on what you can't have, you will feel miserable and deprived. You are reading this book for a reason. You probably feel that something needs to change and you might be ready to change it. What are you moving towards? What drives your healthier decisions? What is it you want? Focusing on those things makes the challenge feel desirable, stokes your motivation and helps you clarify whether you are really ready to make a change.

get to know you

Awareness is the first step in change. Get to know yourself: what hunger feels like, what stress feels like, what fatigue feels like, your daily energy rhythms (when you are most creative, lethargic, energetic, focused, antsy, etc.). Later you can learn to work your day around your rhythms, but if you don't know your rhythms that can be difficult.

Notice what foods give you the most energy for different types of work. A very physically active day may require different foods than a creative planning day. Notice how sleep affects your patience, stress and willpower. Pay attention to which people and activities energize you and which drain you.

You will later be able to use this information as you plan ahead. When you see what kinds of days you have coming up you can best prepare yourself for maximum productivity and enjoyment.

60

Learn to decipher your body's subtle messages. Pay attention to what it is telling you.

learning vs. re-learning

Part of the wellness journey will be learning to listen to and trust your body… again. We instinctively knew a lot of this as small children. We ate when we were hungry and stopped when we were full. We slept when tired and woke when rested. We screamed when we were stressed, played when we needed to.

Our bodies are innately wise and often will tell us what they need…but we have taught ourselves not to listen. As babies and small children we listened to our bodies. We then learned to ignore and override our body's messages and keep eating beyond satiety, to stay up late and get up early to fit more into each day, and to stifle our urge to release stress. Many of us today do not even recognize the feeling of hunger and have not felt well rested in longer than we can remember. We have become so accustomed to feeling overwhelmed and frazzled that we can't remember NOT feeling this way.

So, many of these skills are not brand new to us, we already know them but they are buried. We just need to slow down and listen for our bodies to communicate them to us. We need to trust that we can follow our bodies' needs again. We did it before, we can do it again. We do not need to start from scratch; we just need to uncover an old skill.

• • • •

Our mindset is the foundation on which we build our new lifestyle. Everything from our thoughts to hope, self-compassion to a sense of control, using reminders to pre-planning, and recognizing strengths and alternate truths all affect how easily we can make changes.

3

time management

Time management is important in a discussion of wellness because it is so often our excuse for not doing things. We don't eat well or often enough, sleep enough, exercise, relax or see friends because we "don't have time." We all get 24 hours each day. It boils down to how you choose to spend your time. You can choose to watch TV or get 30 more minutes of sleep, to get up and cook breakfast and pack a lunch or skip breakfast and get a takeout lunch. It is your choice to watch TV or exercise. You can choose to meet your friends for drinks after work or take a class. It is up to you whether you sit and ruminate about an argument rather than do a relaxation exercise.

We are taught to tell time as kids, but not how to manage time. Rarely do we even know how long it takes us to do routine tasks like showering and getting dressed, making dinner, or walking around the block.

We rush through our days not fully aware of how we are spending time and not consciously choosing how to spend our time. We do the same things over and over out of habit, until it feels normal to rush around all day then collapse on the couch with a bag of chips or our two best friends, Ben and Jerry.

create time

We don't "find" extra time; we create it. We can find little pockets of time but we create bigger chunks of time by consolidating and rearranging activities then adding several small pockets of time together. Too often we sit around waiting for time to tap us on the shoulder and say "Here I am, go exercise now."

I suggest keeping a 15-minute increment time log for three days (include at least one weekday and one weekend day) to see exactly what you do with your 24 hours. Every 15 minutes note what you spent most of that time doing. Tracking your time will show you how you spend your time. Wasted time is time not spent working toward a desired outcome. Time well spent is moving you toward a goal or desired outcome. As you review your time logs you will see where you waste time and where you could save time.

If you spend time moving toward your goal you will get there. If you choose to spend time in ways that do not move you forward you will not get there. How do you choose to spend your time?

> "We don't magically find more time, we create it."
>
> Laura Crooks

chunking time

Chunk or batch your time and activities whenever possible. If you need to chop onions for dinner tonight and know you will need chopped onions again tomorrow night, chop them all at once and save half. You save the prep and clean up time by doing it once. If you make roasted chicken tonight, plan to use the extra in enchiladas two nights from now.

If you have three packages to mail, you would not make three separate trips in the same day to mail them; you would take them all at once to save time getting there and waiting in line. Apply the same principle to email; designate a few times a day to open and respond to emails. Responding to each email as they come in means you stop another activity, shift your focus and then have to refocus on the original activity. Refocusing takes, on average, between 10-15 minutes. Interruptions and refocusing, besides taking up a lot of time, make you more prone to accidents or errors.

Reviewing your time log may illuminate just how long you spend mindlessly lost, surfing the Internet. What starts as looking for one piece of information can end several hours later and many videos and articles away from your original plan.

Maybe you can combine activities. There is a time and place for multi-tasking and some things can go well together. Activities using the communication center of your brain, however, do not combine well together; don't try emailing while on a conference call. However, ironing while listening to an audio book or walking and talking with a friend can work well together.

create a time map

Create a 24-hour map of how you would ideally like to spend your time. Block off priority items first; sometimes these are things that take a large chunk of time and sometimes they are things that have a deadline. Fill in smaller time slots with smaller activities. If you fill a bucket with golf balls, then marbles then sand then water you can fit more in than by filling the bucket with sand first, then marbles, then water and you find there is no room for golf balls. Work around your "big" items first.

I think getting enough sleep is so important to all areas of our lives it should be given first dibs on time. Carve out enough hours for sleep so you can feel your best. This might require you asking, "What needs to go so I can get enough sleep?" The next day you can make a different decision. Perhaps the thing you cut today gets priority to-morrow. Maybe you have a party with friends coming up so you are willing to pare down social activities a few days before. If you feel like you did not get enough exer-cise the previous week you can make a point to fit that in this week and spend less time doing something else.

• • • •

Managing time does not need to be static. You are mak-ing decisions with new information over and over during each day and week, fitting things in and weeding things out. Your goal is to eventually spend enough time on each activity to be working toward meeting your goal.

4

stress management

Managing stress is the linchpin in our wellness. Stress affects our choice of foods, how well we metabolize what we eat, and how we store fat. Our sleep, happiness, mood, energy level, and exercise are also affected by stress. Exercise can reduce stress, but when we are stressed we often choose to skip exercising. We might turn to comfort foods and overeating, which further stress us.

Stress can aggravate most diseases and conditions, from cardiovascular disease to memory, from infertility to digestive disorders. Stress changes our bodies neuro-chemically and hormonally. Learning to manage stress plays a huge role in our wellness. I will share two primary ways of managing stress: physically relaxing your mind and body, and mentally changing your perspective so that you don't perceive as much as being stressful.

stress is

Stress is our response to situations that we perceive are beyond our ability to handle. It is our perception of an event and our belief that we don't have the skills to manage it. When we encounter stress our body sends a series of hormones and neurochemicals to activate the sympathetic nervous system, which prepares us for a fight or flight. Our hearts race, our breathing deepens, our muscles tense, blood flow is diverted from digestion to our skeletal muscles so we are prepared to run or evade danger. This response is helpful in the event of an animal attack, but how often do we really need to fend off wild animals? Often our "attacks" are perceived slights from a coworker, the rudeness of other drivers, hunger, fatigue, pain, a checkbook that doesn't balance, or inconsiderate behavior from sales people. Our stress is rarely from situations requiring a physical escape.

Stress is not all bad. We need some stress, but most of us have more than we need. Stress helps us get out of bed each morning and meet deadlines. The problem arises from the amount of stress we have in our lives and our inability to manage it.

stress response

Stress can be physical, mental or emotional. Your body responds the same regardless of the source. Stress can be acute (such as with random, sudden events like the washing machine overflowing or a car accident) or chronic (regular and predictable annoyances like irritating co-workers, daily traffic, skipping meals and overbooked schedules). Your body responds the same way to acute stress as it does to chronic stress.

Adrenaline and cortisol, the two most widely known stress hormones, prepare your body for action. Adrenaline causes your heart to beat faster and cortisol affects how your blood sugar and insulin are utilized in trying to fuel your body. These hormonal effects affect your sleep, food choices, metabolism, energy, and blood sugar levels, which all affect your health and wellness.

acute and chronic stress

Acute stressors can be good or bad things and include getting married or divorced, an illness, a traffic ticket, get-ting a promotion, moving, having children, and losing a job. Chronic stressors can include finances, relatives, poor food choices, lack of sleep, chronic illnesses, care-giving, rude people, phone trees, overbooked appoint-ments, negativity, a non-supportive relationship, clutter, frustration, and endless amounts of household chores.

With acute stress, once the event is over our body starts settling back down and hormones return to their normal levels. With chronic stress, our stressors are layered and overlap each other, causing our neurochemicals to stay elevated, never having the chance to subside. It is the chronic stress that ruins our health.

The newer branch of medicine called psychoneuroimmu-nology studies the interactions between the body and brain and how our immune and nervous systems are af-fected by our behaviors. Our hormones, neurochemicals and immune system are all altered by stress.

real or imagined

Because of your powerful mind-body connection, your body responds the same way whether your stress is real or imagined: "I am late for my job interview" and "What if I am late for my job interview, don't get the job and become homeless?" trigger the same response. Your body also responds the same way to a current event as it does to you rehashing a past event. "I am so angry that this person just insulted me" and "I remember when so and so insulted me 10 years ago and I can still feel that anger" can warrant the same response. If your brain is spending time on an issue, your body steps in to help resolve it. Your brain cannot distinguish between real events and thoughts or memories; they both trigger a physiological response.

fluidity of stress

Some situations may always affect us more than others but over time the things that stress us change because our coping skills and experiences change. Things that scared or overwhelmed you in your teens may not bother you in your 30s. You have encountered a lot in that time and acquired new skills. What bothers you today may not be an issue next year. Managing stress is a skill and you do improve with practice. Once you have handled a crisis, a similar event will not be as stressful because you have the experience of coping with it.

The state of your body also affects how well you handle stress. How you eat, sleep, exercise and handle your emotions affect your stress. You have probably recognized that you are more irritable and less patient when tired or hungry. When your stress accumulates and you don't provide an outlet or make time for relaxation, very small things may set you off. Poor, non-nutritious food choices contribute to you handling stress less well. So you can be sure the weeks when you run yourself ragged (working late, eating junk, not sleeping enough, not having fun) are taking a toll and you will feel more stress.

what stress feels like

We each feel our stress differently but there are similarities we all share. Chronic stress can affect every system of the body from our heads to our toes. You may notice forgetfulness, irritability, depression, anxiety, crying, moodiness, hair loss, twitches, high-pitched voice, nervous laughter, headaches, muscle tension, increased pain, rapid breathing, chest tightness, rapid heartbeat, heart palpitations, high blood pressure, clammy hands, increased sweating, weakened immune system and susceptibility to illness, less saliva and more tooth decay, abdominal cramps, diarrhea, constipation, poor digestion, food cravings, weight gain or weight loss, fluttery or heavy sensation in stomach, infertility, osteoporosis, weak or brittle hair and nails, poor wound healing, and flare ups of skin conditions such as herpes simplex, psoriasis or acne.

Knowing your stressors and learning to anticipate stress-ful situations lets you plan ahead either by doing more relaxation exercises to better handle the stress or by making changes that minimize the stress or your re-sponse to it. What people, places, or situations trigger your stress? Do holidays, loud gatherings, or certain peo-ple routinely bother you? Knowing this beforehand gives you some power.

Learn to recognize your personal symptoms of stress so you can notice your stress early and head it off. Do you feel stress primarily in your mood, a lack of creativity and patience, in your muscles, or your stomach or bowels? Tune into the earliest signs and have more time to make a plan for handling that stress.

The way the mind and body are connected means that we can get ourselves riled up and calmed down by the thoughts we have. Thinking of something horrible and thinking of something special and beautiful will cause 2 different responses in your body. Thinking positive, loving thoughts can calm your nervous system (think in detail about a pet you love, a favorite vacation spot, doing a hobby). You can calm yourself by actually being with your pet or by clearly imagining being with your pet.

relaxation

Relaxation is not the same as relaxing your body, which is why your mind can race when you go to bed. Relaxation is intentionally focusing your mind on one thing; it is focused, active, and purposeful. Lying in front of the TV, using drugs or alcohol or food to block out emotions is not relaxation. Zoning out, walling off or avoiding feeling emotions is not relaxing. Instead, find something you can completely focus on for even a short amount of time. Having your mind focused and not thinking 400 things at once is calming to your nervous system.

mindfulness

In doing something mindfully, doing just one thing with full attention, you can engage your parasympathetic nervous system, which promotes relaxation, healing, growth, creativity and productivity. You are also quieting your sympathetic nervous system, the famed fight-or-flight response, which elevates your blood pressure, heart rate, cortisol levels, and feelings of rage.

Mindfulness means slowing down and focusing all of your senses on one thing. If you are brushing your teeth mind- fully you think only about brushing your teeth, feeling the toothpaste and toothbrush, tasting and smelling the tooth- paste. You see and feel the foam build, see and feel it as you spit it out. You are not walking around picking out clothing and making your bed while you brush. You aren't even planning your day. You are simply brushing your teeth and noticing yourself brushing.

Pick things you already do each day and choose to do them or part of them mindfully. You can eat a meal (or the first three bites) mindfully. You can shower, cook, wash your hands, iron, sit outside, or enter your car mindfully. Pay attention to the details of what you are doing.

Mindfulness is the opposite of multitasking. Mindfulness is being present and engaged while doing something. The mental to-do list can wait two minutes while you enjoy the feeling of finishing one small activity being fully present. We often don't have a beginning and ending to activities because we are doing four things simultaneously and while one ends we are still plowing through the others and do not have the sense of closure.

Washing your hair is part of showering, but if you single out washing your hair and zoom in to only focus on that (the sensations, smell, texture, temperature, the water, the sounds...) it can be very relaxing to your nervous system to have the awareness of completion of that one task, even though it is part of a larger task. Think about what you can do mindfully. Remind yourself to do it mindfully and enjoy the slowness of it!

breathing

Taking four slow, full belly breaths (breathing in through the nose, pause, and exhaling gently, slowly and fully either through your nose or mouth) is one of the quickest and easiest ways to start calming your nervous system. Direct your breath down toward your belly, not up into your shoulders. Feel your breath, feel your chest and belly expand and contract. And make your exhale longer than your inhale.

Schedule times during the day to breathe like this. I use red lights as my reminder and use those moments to focus on my breathing. You can use anything you do repeatedly during the day as your reminder to breathe mindfully: walking through a certain doorway, washing your hands, eating. Don't feel weird about having to re-mind yourself to relax. Use notes, alarms, and routine activities to establish this new habit.

ways to relax

Many people say they don't have time to re-lax but you can start in as little as two minutes.

You can begin to feel your heart rate slow down, your muscles relax, and your mind become quiet in just moments.

Try allowing yourself two minutes a day to unwind by doing one of the following very

Four slow, full belly breaths is one of the quickest ways to start calming your nervous system.

1. Inhale slowly and gently through your nose feeling your chest and belly expand
2. Pause
3. Then gently and fully let your breath out either through your nose or mouth, feeling your chest and belly contract.

Focus on the sensations of your breath flowing in and out.

consciously and purposefully. Your mind will wander. Just bring it back and keep going. For some of these ideas,

closing your eyes might help you focus by minimizing dis-
tractions. You could:

- sip tea

- watch the clouds or a candle flame

- imagine a wonderful vacation in detail (engage as
  many senses as possible in envisioning your special
  place – the fragrance, temperature, colors, textures,
  sounds…)

- swing or rock in a rocking chair

- massage your feet or hands

- stretch

- listen to music, chimes or nature sounds

- rub a polished stone

- play with dry rice

- follow your breathing

- write in a gratitude journal

Relaxing is a skill, the more you practice the better you
get. Your mind will wander less and less the more you do

it. With experience you will begin to enter a relaxed state more easily and quickly.

You can put technology to use in managing your stress; there are apps for stress management. Some have chimes, timers, reminders, guided imageries or nature sounds. Or you can program your phone to sound peri-odically to remind you to take a few minutes to relax and unwind.

Relax in 2 minutes. Do something mindfully, being fully present and aware:

- wash your hands
- stretch and relax a rubber band between your fingers
- roll your feet over a golf ball
- sit outside with your eyes closed and listen to the sounds of nature

changing your perspective

In addition to encouraging your mind and body to slow down, you can change the way you choose to respond to stressful events. Changing your perspective or being able to see another view is commonly called re-framing. This is not meant to ignore what is happening; you still feel the emotions as necessary, but you move through the negative ones instead of getting trapped in them.

Can you consciously look for another perspective to the situation bothering you? Can you change the emotions you attach to the event? How might someone else see it? Could there be a backstory you aren't aware of? Could the person who talks too loudly be hard of hearing? Might the person tailgating or cutting your off in traffic be rushing to the hospital to find their loved one? Could the person who doesn't leave you alone really just like your company a lot? Could the traffic jam give you the opportunity to listen to your favorite song again or hear more of your audio book? What is another way to view the problem?

4As

A technique I especially like is called the "4 As": avoid, accept, adapt and alter. This technique requires you to be creative in how you think about and respond to things that stress you.

avoid

Are you able to avoid the person, place or thing that causes you stress? Sometimes you can and sometimes you can't. If you can't totally avoid it or them, can you minimize contact with it/them? It could be a store, a road, a person, or a type of gathering. There are probably ways you can work around it.

There was a particular store that I just didn't like, but for some reason still shopped there occasionally. I did not like the store layout, the employees, the smell, the lighting, the other shoppers...nothing. Then it dawned on me – I don't have to shop there. I haven't been back!

accept

Are you able to simply accept that what is bothering you is bothering you? Let's say you find yourself in an unexpected traffic jam and you will be late. You have the choice of clenching the steering wheel and swearing and getting angry or you can take a breath and accept that you will be late and choose to stay calm. Staying frustrated will not get you there any sooner, but you will arrive frantic and angry and unable to focus. By accepting the situation for what it is you could experience less stress.

adapt

Adapting is changing your mindset about the event. Maybe you can't avoid a stressor and you aren't going to accept it, but can you adapt to it? Can you shore up your inner strength and make the best of a holiday meal with that family? Can the longer commute to a new job be time to learn a language in the car?

alter

Sometimes we can't totally change a stressful situation but we can change it a little. Instead of spending four days with relatives at their house maybe you could alter it and stay in a hotel, or cut the trip to two days. Move your meetings with people who get off topic to a neutral place so that you can get up and leave when you have finished discussing business. Can you take a different route to work or shift your work time to avoid traffic?

find the humor

Similar to shifting your perspective is to find the humorous angle. You are shifting the perspective specifically to the funny slant. You might not think something is funny now, but could you see how it might seem funny in the future? Think about whether any sitcom or comedian would be able to use the material for a skit. Laughter can lower your stress.

will it matter in a year

We get so caught up in the event that all we can't see the forest for the trees. All we see is the bad in our stressful event. Let's say you arrive at work with two similar but different shoes on, or you find baby vomit on your collar. While this is stressful when you discover your fashion faux pas, will it really matter in a year? How many people do you really think will remember or care in a week?

build your stress management toolbox

Having a selection of stress management tools is essential. There will be certain times and places that a particular technique works well and other situations when that technique won't be practical. I find petting my rabbits, working in my garden, and watching a lava lamp particularly relaxing. But these techniques are not portable;

Manage your stress:
- know your stressors
- avoid or minimize those you can
- create a relaxation practice
- know which types of relaxation exercises you do and do not like

85

I can't use them in traffic or during a meeting. I often am able to fit in a few stretches or do a visualization exercise anywhere and I can always simply follow my breath or try to find humor in the situation.

You won't like all types of relaxation techniques and that's OK. But if you don't experiment with many types you won't discover all the forms that you do like. A few to try include: progressive muscle relaxation, visualization, guided imagery, biofeedback, meditation, yoga, prayer, massage, Reiki, reflexology, becoming still and quiet with a mantra, stretching, playing music, tai chi or art therapy. You may like to be guided through a relaxation exercise or prefer doing it your own way. Both are right and the best way is the way that works best for you!

Knowing a variety of ways to change your perspective is another way to add tools to your stress management tool-box. Seeing a situation from another viewpoint can help us let go of some stress.

• • • •

Know what causes your stress and do what you can to change it. Practice relaxation exercises both regularly and in the moment. Work on accepting and changing what you can and trying to see stressful events from all angles.

Managing your stress will improve your sleep and energy levels, you will have more control over your eating, your metabolism should improve, and your patience, mood and creativity will improve, also. You will feel better when you control the stress in your life and your response to it.

5

eating

The food you choose to eat affects how you feel and function. You are at your best when eating appropriate amounts of healthy foods. When you have enough quality gas in your tank you run better. When you fill up on nutritionally poor foods it is like starving your body. Digesting junky food leaves you fatigued, cranky, fat and with inflammation. In a word: stressed. Eating poor quality food and not eating enough food causes stress in your body. Food, both quantity and quality, affects our sleep, stress, energy level, mood, creativity and productivity.

what, why, how

When we think about eating we often jump to *what* we should eat. In considering which specific foods to eat you also need to consider which not to eat. While our food choices are important, so are the reasons *why* we eat and *how* we eat.

what we eat

Good quality, nutritious foods give us energy. Poor food choices drain our energy and can lead to inflammation and chronic diseases. It would be unrealistic to think that every morsel of food we eat is 100% good for us. In general, we benefit from eating real food and less refined, processed food.

healthy eating

There is no one right way to eat. We are all different and our metabolic needs change over time. While many people want to eat a healthier diet, this can mean something different to everyone. Eating healthier depends on what you currently eat.

Healthy eating could mean increasing:

- fiber
- antioxidants
- variety
- nutrients
- omega-3 fats
- fruits and vegetables

- meal planning
- cooking at home
- food quality

It could also mean decreasing:

- calories
- portion sizes
- processed foods
- fats
- sugar
- mindless munching
- restaurant food
- refined carbs
- emotional eating

Healthy eating could also mean:

- getting enough calories
- eating breakfast
- eating often enough

- making better snack choices
- balancing protein with vegetables and fruits
- sitting at a table to eat
- eating mindfully or purposefully
- improving the quality of your food
- eating sustainably
- eating organic
- eating only when hungry
- eating locally and seasonally
- eating less food overall

Healthy eating is a flexible concept. Get very specific about what it means to you. After you clarify your definition of healthy eating, determine some small steps you can take this week. For example: eating more vegetables might mean you start by going to the grocery store to notice all the vegetable options. Then you might need to research recipes: ask friends, do an Internet search, read cookbooks. This is all before you even buy a new vegetable. And you may need to try it several times and prepared several different ways before you officially decide to like it or not.

It is often easier to add a new healthier food in than to take out a frequent comfort food. Try adding a healthier food and eating it first. As you start to pay attention to your hunger you will be able to stop eating before you get to the less healthy food and it will naturally be decreased or eliminated. Also, the food you eat first can become your anchor food and set the tone for the meal, prompting you to make better subsequent food choices.

How you spend your day also affects what you should eat. Very active days require more calories than seden-tary days. You may find more protein on active days keeps you energized. Or you may feel best with smaller but more frequent meals of complex carbohydrates (like fruit or vegetables). Get to know your body, your rhythms and needs.

why we eat

Ideally we eat because we are hungry and we enjoy the food we eat. However, hunger is one of the last reasons we eat. We often find ourselves eating because food is available (samples in stores, candy on a coworker's desk, nuts at the bar, bread basket at the restaurant…), be-cause it is time to eat (it's noon, this is when someone can relieve you for lunch, dinner is served...), due to emotions (we might be sad, bored, nervous, angry...), we eat so as not to offend someone (a loved one cooked for us or wants to see us eat seconds...), because we saw or smelled food or are somewhere we associate with food (movies, the bakery smell at the grocery store, the food court at the mall, fast food on the way to the soccer field...), or for celebrations (alcohol and cake seem to have prominent roles in celebrations).

Many people do not know the feeling of hunger. Try letting yourself get hungry so you can really feel hunger. Notice your personal symptoms. Do you feel weak, light headed, cranky, unfocused, or jittery? Does your stomach rumble? Do you get a headache?

Feeling some hunger is not an emergency. Most of us have access to food within a matter of minutes if not seconds, even when we are in our cars. Our bodies are designed to give us hunger warning signals and we can withstand some hunger.

Learn to predict about when you might get hungry based on what and when you last ate and what you have done since you last ate. Plan your meals and snacks based on what you need and when you need it.

how we eat

Why should you pay attention to how you eat? Because how you eat affects your enjoyment of food, how much you eat, what you eat, your weight, your digestion, and your health.

Imagine an ideal dining experience: the location, the sounds, the aromas. What makes it wonderful? Is it relaxed, peaceful and fun? It might include a quiet setting, a table with dishes, utensils and cloth napkins. There might be music, soft lighting, and pleasant conversation. There is probably delicious food (maybe even cooked and cleared by someone else!).

Now picture your average meal. Is it more rushed or chaotic than your ideal? Are you even sitting at a table eating from a plate? Are your surroundings conducive to enjoying a meal? Did you notice your food? Did you taste what you ate? Did you even want to taste it?

We are surrounded by messages from the media and marketers encouraging us to eat (and overeat) quickly and on the go. The faster we eat, the more we buy. Think about the words marketers use to describe eating: grab, gulp, slurp, guzzle, "pound them down," slam, fast, instant, quick, and convenient. They sound like words from a fraternity party gone bad, not descriptions of a meal. Those words all convey action and imply that we are so busy we need to cram food in on the go.

Foods are now designed to be eaten with one hand (so we can drive or type with the other hand?), are precooked and served (sold) in a disposable wrapper. It's all so frantic. It is not a coincidence that the number of Americans who eat while driving has increased as the number of foods made to be eaten with one hand increased.

Eating is about more than just refueling. It should be a pleasurable experience, one that lets you slow down and involve all of your senses. Food should nourish your soul as well as your body. Savor, sip, taste, enjoy, experience, delicious, linger, flavor are words that should describe eating, even if you eat alone. Let yourself taste the food and follow your body's signal of when you have eaten enough.

You can start to shift your eating experience by taking a deep breath, sitting down with your food on a plate and noticing what you will be eating. Take time to chew, taste and appreciate each bite.

Create one meal a day or one meal a week where you can take the time to slow down and enjoy what you eat. Make time for a meal without any gulping, guzzling or steering wheels.

mindful eating

It may seem awkward but try taking a few extra minutes to eat something mindfully. Really slow down the process of eating and enjoying your food.

Anticipate enjoying the food.

Think about what it reminds you of: people, occasions, emotions, etc.

Imagine what you think it will taste like.

Appreciate how the food got to you, where it was grown, the people involved.

Look at your food, noticing the colors and textures.

97

Inhale the aroma of your food.

If appropriate, feel the weight of it and the textures.

Take one bite and without chewing it feel it in your mouth.

Notice the flavor and textures.

Chew the bite and swallow.

Put down your utensil and think about how you just ate one bite of food.

Take another moment to savor the texture and flavor and experience of your food.

hunger scale

Try using a hunger scale to help you eat only when you are hungry. Think of your hunger on a 1-10 scale with 1 being extremely hungry and 10 being painfully full. When you are too hungry you make poor food choices and go for whatever is fast and easy. These choices are often sold in vending machines, are high in calories, sugar and fat, and low in nutrients. When we are very hungry we slip into food emergency mode and our goal is to eat anything so that we don't feel hungry anymore.

Try to stay away from the end zones of the hunger scale. Eat when you are at about a 3 and stop when you are at about a 7. At a 3 you still have enough control to take a few minutes to make a healthier selection. Stopping at 7 you are satisfied but not stuffed. Your body can function well without the discomfort of a bulging stomach.

Each time you are about to eat, ask yourself why you are reaching for food. If the answer is not hunger then do something else. Try distracting yourself for at least 10 minutes and often the non-hunger urge to eat passes.

● ● ● ●

Eating affects your wellness, your energy level, your stress, your sleep and your mood. We should be eating mindfully, for hunger and with enjoyment. Pay attention to how, what and why you eat.

Tips for better eating:

Define what you want to change about your eating. Your desired outcome and your current status will help you decide where you are, where you are going and what you need to do to get there. The following tips have helped people make improvements in their eating habits.

- plan ahead
- eliminate decision points
    - eat the same breakfast or lunch daily
    - plan meals a few days ahead
    - decide what to order before arriving at the restaurant
- keep a list of favorite or go-to meals
- keep a few staple ingredients on hand
- prep and cook once, eat twice
- clear the kitchen clutter
- clear the counters
- arrange the cupboards so they are functional and useful
- invest in knives you enjoy using
- keep healthier foods visible, keep treats out of sight
- establish set meal times
- establish set snacks
- eat breakfast

- combine protein (a small amount will do) with all meals/ snacks
- never shop when hungry
- use smaller plates
- eat slowly
- create an end of meal ritual
- create an eating-only zone (no clutter)
- serve from the stove (but put fruits and green vegetables on the table)
- fill half your plate with non-starchy vegetables
- serve 3/4 your usual portion. If you are still hungry after 20 minutes have a bit more

6

sleep

Sleep is vital to our wellness. Sleep affects our mood, patience, stress, food choices, appetite, satiety, energy levels, growth, healing, tissue repair, happiness, and our propensity to exercise.

Sleep is crucial for managing our stress. When well rested we have more patience, tolerance, creativity and productivity. We also have more energy and are more likely to exercise and prepare nutritious foods. During sleep our appetite hormones reset; when we have not slept enough we tend to feel hungrier all day and less satisfied when we do eat. Our stress hormones cause us to crave sweet and fatty foods.

It is still not known exactly why we need to sleep but we definitely need it. (Maybe after thinking our 60,000 thoughts each day we are simply tired!) During sleep our bodies rest, grow and repair. Our brain is active during sleep processing and storing memories and experiences.

how much

We all need sleep, and most Americans need more than what they are getting. Most adults need 7-9 hours of sleep nightly to function optimally. Many people say they do just fine with only five hours and while there are some people who truly function well on five or six hours of sleep, most of us perform better with more than that. You are getting enough sleep when you wake up without an alarm clock and feel refreshed. If you struggle at the sound of an alarm clock try getting more sleep for several nights and see how you feel.

sabotaging our sleep

Our lifestyle can inhibit good sleep. Going to bed too full or too hungry can make sleep difficult. Both alcohol and the TV being on can prevent us from reaching the deeper, restorative levels of sleep. Not getting enough exercise can make it harder to fall asleep as can anxiety and mental clutter. Caffeine and drinking too much of anything too close to bedtime can wake us up for a trip to the bathroom. Pets in the bedroom, especially in the bed, can be disruptive. Snoring and sleep apnea, either yours or your partner's, can also ruin a good night's rest.

Then we have the ever popular habit of staying up to finish one more thing and/or getting up early to fit just a bit more into our day. We don't even give ourselves enough time in bed with the lights out to get enough sleep.

creating closure

Our brains are like files, we can only have so many open at once before we create a mess and lose things. We only hold 7-10 pieces of information in our short-term memory. If we can get things out of our mind we can stop trying to remember them. Try making a list on paper or in your phone. Then tell yourself that it is safely recorded and you can move on.

Often times we can't fall asleep because our minds are whirring along. If we don't have closure it is like leaving the files open, ready to be worked on. When our brains are full we don't feel like we are at the end of a cycle or in a place to stop. One way to "close a file" is to create closure rituals. Following the same routine at the end of an activity lets your body know you are done with that activity. You can close out a meal, a project, your workday, or your day in general. Creating a bedtime ritual is one more way of telling your body and mind it is time to slow down and prepare for sleep. Do a final task mindfully, noting when your day is done.

worrying

Make a list of the things worrying you. Getting them out of your mind allows your brain to rest so you can sleep. For some people establishing a set worry time can help. Pick 15 minutes in the afternoon or early evening that becomes your worry time. During that time do all of your worrying and nothing else. Time is up either after 15 minutes or when you start thinking about things other than your worries. If you did not get to worry about everything, write the remaining worries down so you can start with them tomorrow. If worries arise outside of worry time add them to a list but do not dwell on them until worry time. While this may sound crazy it works well for many people. By having a contained time and place for worrying our mind can relax knowing we have a time dedicated to it, it is not left hanging as an open file in our mind.

scheduling sleep

Sleep should be the first thing you schedule in your 24-hour day. Start with the time you need to get up, and work backwards, blocking off the amount of time you need to be asleep to feel well. This is your sleep time. Next add on however many minutes it takes you to get ready to get into bed. This can include picking an outfit for the next day, brushing your teeth, locking the doors, reading in bed and all the time it takes you to settle into bed in order to fall asleep. Now block off your "getting ready to go to sleep" time.

So if I want to get eight hours of sleep (meaning I want to *sleep* a full eight hours) and I need to wake up at 7 AM, I need to be asleep by 11 PM. If it takes me 20 minutes to read in bed then fall asleep I need to be in bed by 10:40 PM. If it takes me 20 minutes to wash my face, brush my teeth, and get undressed I need to start that process at 10:20 PM.

I need to honestly know how long it takes me to get to my bedroom once I say I am going to bed. If I need 30 minutes because I always stop to hang up a coat, put three more plates in the dishwasher, wipe the counters and get the bunnies ready for the night, then I need to start "going to bed" at 9:50 PM. So now getting eight hours of sleep and going to sleep at 11 PM means I start heading upstairs at 9:50 PM. I need to think of my "getting ready for bed" time as 9:50, not 11.

In the 30-60 minutes leading up to my "getting ready for bed" time I start winding down and get ready to get ready for bed.

Sleep hygiene and bedtime should be a priority all day. Plan your day and budget your time so that you can get eight hours of sleep. This might mean watching how much fluid you drink in the evening (so that you do not have to get up to use the bathroom). It means thinking about when to cut off caffeine. This could be after 7 PM or after 10 AM depending on how you respond to caffeine. Consider what foods might cause heartburn or indigestion, what movies might cause nightmares, and how to create a relaxing environment leading up to bedtime.

sleep hygiene

during the day:

- Do your worrying well before bedtime.

- Doing a relaxation exercise at some point during the day can enhance your sleep.

- Get out in morning light.

- Get physical activity.

- Limit daytime naps, too long or too late in the day and they may interfere with your night's sleep.

in the 30-60 minutes before bed:

- Have a routine leading up to bedtime.

- Dim the lights.

- Do something relaxing, repetitive or calming: stretches, reading for pleasure, listening to soothing music, a pastime that does not require sharp thinking or strong emotions.

- Avoid screens (computer, TV, phones, tablets…). The lights from these stimulate our brain neurons.

- Taking a bath or shower at bedtime can help you un- wind and fall asleep. The heat of the shower/bath raises your body temperature, then as you cool off you get tired. Your body temperature naturally drops a bit at bedtime. The shower/bath can accentuate that.

- Limit alcohol. While a drink might make us feel re-laxed and two drinks might make us sleepy, sleep af-ter alcohol is not restful. You may fall asleep easily but you do not progress into deeper levels of sleep so you do not wake up feeling refreshed.

- Avoid big heavy or spicy meals just before bed. Too much food or spicy food can lead to heartburn when you lie down.

in bed:

- Keep the bedroom dark (avoid lights from appliances, chargers....especially blue ones. Either remove them, cover them or turn them toward the wall so the light does not disturb your sleep)

- Consider using white noise like a fan or nature sound machine to provide a soothing steady noise, espe-cially to block out irritating or sporadic noises such as snoring or household noises.

- No pets in the bedroom. They wake you up with noises and movement.

- Keep the room cool. We sleep most soundly when the room is comfortably cool. If you feel cold, wear socks or a sweatshirt to bed.

- If you use an alarm clock, set it for the time you need to get up and do not use the snooze button. Snoozing for nine minutes does not let you fall into a deep enough sleep to refresh you.

- Keep a fairly stable sleep and wake up time even on the weekends.

- If you wake up with a sore back or stiff neck consider replacing your mattress or pillows. Neither lasts for-ever!

waking during the night

If you wake during the night try a relaxation exercise to get back to sleep (follow your breathing, or become aware of each body part, one at a time,

sleep hygiene includes:

- creating a cool dark room
- eliminating disturbances in the bedroom (like pets, TVs, and charging lights)
- create a winding down routine
- consider using a white noise sound
- keep a stable bedtime and wake up time

from your toes to your head, or try relaxing one body part at a time)

If you wake up about the same time most nights to go to the bathroom, decide whether you really have to go to the bathroom or you just get up to go because there seems to be nothing else to do and that has become your habit. Try staying in bed and doing a relaxation exercise instead to unlearn the habit of using the bathroom. Then work on unlearning the habit of waking up during the night. Teach yourself to stay in bed, asleep.

medical reasons

Our weight impacts our sleep. Carrying excess weight, especially around the neck, can cause snoring and sleep apnea. Having a large belly, especially a full one, can cause gastric reflux when we lie down.

There can be medical reasons (diseases, medications) for not getting a good night's sleep and your health care provider can review them with you. But often our sleep and our routines leading up to sleep become habitual and inhibit our sleep. Getting enough sleep should be a priority.

• • • •

Sleep is truly vital to our health and wellness yet we rarely get enough. With enough sleep we can better control our appetites and make better food choices, boost our energy and mood, reduce our stress and have a better chance of getting a good workout. Getting adequate sleep lets us work with our bodies instead of fighting against ourselves.

7

exercise

Our bodies are designed to move, and exercise is really just movement. Without continued use of our joints and muscles we will lose strength, flexibility and eventually mobility. Exercise can improve our digestion, mood, metabolism, stress, eating, happiness, sleep and willpower.

Exercise is known to improve our mood; it can help combat anxiety and depression as well as boost our happiness and make us feel better. It does not have to be an hour-long run to create the famed "runners high" and endorphin release. Short bursts of mild activity help, too.

Regular activity helps keep our metabolism humming along and keeps our gastrointestinal system moving as well. Regular exercisers may find themselves making better food choices to match their commitment to exercise.

Our sleep is enhanced when we move daily. The newer research is refuting the old adage that you shouldn't do strenuous cardio just before bed because it delays sleep.

While this may be true for some people, it is certainly not true for everyone.

Exercise can be a great stress reliever. It can be a way to blow off steam or create a calming, rhythmic action. When your stress is better managed you make better food choices, you sleep better and your mood is better. Exercising outside can be especially relaxing.

Exercise was an integral part of our ancestors' day and today we develop gadgets and procedures so that we need to move less (remote controls, online shopping, takeout delivery, etc.). So now we spend our days less active than ever and then try to fit in some exercise.

inactivity

It is currently believed that inactivity might be the biggest threat to our health. Even people who exercise generally still spend enough time sitting to be detrimental to their health. Time spent purposefully exercising is simply not enough to undo the hazards of several hours of inactivity. There are health benefits to being active and we now know there are health risks to being inactive.

Our days may be busy, but they are generally not active. We sit during commutes, sit in meetings, sit at our desks, sit waiting for appointments and then sit for enjoyment such as movies or ballgames. Think about how you can move for even five minutes every hour. Can you set an alarm to remind you to stand up and move around periodically? Can you take phone calls standing or marching in place? Can you take the stairs instead of the elevator for even one flight? Can you do ten jumping jacks between meetings or activities? Avoiding or breaking long periods of inactivity will help your health and wellness.

benefits

The benefits of exercise are numerous, but still not enough to get some people moving. For many people not exercising is a habit, and a hard one to change. Exercise improves your

Break up periods of inactivity:
- stand for 2 minutes of every hour
- walk to a water cooler on another floor hourly
- march in place during phone calls or while cooking
- do chair or desk stretches hourly
- tap your feet while answering emails
- do crunches during commercials

117

energy, complexion, metabolism, strength, insulin sensitivity, mood, figure, memory, self-esteem and sleep. It can reshape your body, relieve stress, reduce pain, boost your happiness, and strengthen your lungs and heart. It can help control your weight, blood pressure, blood sugar and cholesterol. There's something for everyone in that list! All this from something that can be free and fun.

components of exercise

There are four components to a well-rounded exercise program: cardiovascular or aerobic activity, strength or resistance training, flexibility or stretching and balance. We all should get some of each, but depending on our goals and body composition how much time we spend doing each will vary.

cardio

Cardio includes sustained movement that raises your heart rate for a continuous period of time and requires oxygen to meet the energy demand. Cardio can be either low impact like swimming, walking, using an elliptical machine, and cycling, which are all easier on the joints, or high impact (when both feet are off the ground at some point) like running, jumping rope or boxing. Plyometric

exercises are a form of high impact exercises that incor-
porate jumping and are good for developing explosive-
ness, speed and power.

Cardio can be done at low or high intensity depending on
how hard you push yourself. You can take a stroll, and
keep your heart rate and breathing low or you can power
walk and accelerate your heart rate and breathing. Similarly, you can jog, swim or cycle at a relaxed pace or at a
sprint. Cardio can be relaxing and calming especially at
lower intensities; the steady rhythm of movement can be
soothing.

Even people who spend all day on their feet may not be
taking many steps (OR nurses, classroom teachers) or
getting an elevated heart rate. So while they have movement built into their day, they still need focused periods of
cardio (aerobic activity).

strength training
Strength training is for everyone, not just big men at the
gym. Women, you will not bulk up from lifting weights.
While it is an integral part of a comprehensive program
you don't need to do it daily. Especially important if lifting
weights to build muscle is to let each muscle group rest 1-

3 days before lifting again. Having strong muscles gives our bodies definition and function and helps protect us from injury. Muscle looks better than fat; it takes up less space and doesn't jiggle. Strength training takes many forms: weight machines, free weights, resistance bands, body weight and what I call "yard items" (ropes and tires) to name a few.

There are different ways to lift and different focuses and theories. A few sessions with a qualified personal trainer can be money well spent. Whether you choose yoga or free weights, definitely work with someone who can show you correct form and who understands your goals. There are trainers who prefer working with bodybuilders and there are trainers who prefer working with people just starting a workout program; pick your trainer to match your needs.

Some forms of exercise can combine cardio and strength training: kettlebells, yoga, Pilates, circuit training, boot camp. The advantages of combining the two include less boredom repeating the same movement over and over, bigger calorie burn in a shorter amount of time, calorie burning continuing after the exercise session ends.

flexibility

Flexibility or stretching keeps your muscles long and supple. As muscles tighten and shorten we lose some range of motion. As we age we need to devote more time to stretching.

balance

Our sense of balance comes from a strong core and fit body. As we age we need to devote more time to improving our balance. You can build balance training in to other activities. Brush your teeth or do bicep curls standing on one leg and do toe raises during phone calls. Yoga can really help your balance.

exercise outcomes

We each have different desired outcomes from exercise: lose weight (burn fat), build muscle, get toned (improve muscle definition), increase strength, improve endurance, ease pain and stiffness, become more flexible and coordinated, or to relax. Our goal affects what type of exercise we do and how we do it. If my goal is to ease arthritis pain and stiffness I will move more gently and focus on mobility more than someone training for a marathon; I may go for three short walks a day and do tai chi. When training for a marathon I need longer periods of exercise for endurance plus time devoted to strength and speed. If your primary goal is to lose weight you will spend more time on cardio and strength training than someone looking to sculpt muscles and improve joint range of motion, who might spend more time on flexibility and strength training.

All four types of exercise benefit all of us but how much of each we do may look very different. Our body type, our goals, our general activity level, our eating, stress and sleep all impact our exercise.

how long

"I don't have time" is such a common excuse for not exercising. You do not have to exercise for an hour or even 30 consecutive minutes to reap benefits. Several 5 or 10-minute segments do add up. (However, if endurance or stamina is your goal you will need long chunks of time.)

Some days you may be able to fit everything in in one longer session. Other days you may need to break your exercise into smaller time chunks.

You can fit more exercise and calorie burning into a shorter amount of time by combining strength and cardio moves and increasing your intensity. Weave one minute of cardio such as jumping rope between each set of lifting weights. The cardio provides the rest for the muscle group being strengthened and the short bursts of cardio mixed in keep your heart rate up.

You can also try exercising at a higher intensity for fewer minutes. Instead of a 3mph walk go the same distance at a faster pace. Or intersperse 30-60 seconds of all out intensity with a pace that lets you catch your breath for 1-3 minutes, and keep repeating this. This is sometimes called interval training or high intensity interval training (HIIT). Repeatedly shifting your effort and intensity from moderate to high can burn more calories in a shorter amount of time.

I hate it

"I hate to sweat" is another common complaint. This complaint can be lessened by timing when you exercise. If you exercise in the middle of the day, showering and re-doing hair and makeup can be time consuming. But if you time your exercise for the beginning or end of your day you can shower once and be done. When you feel like you can sweat like a beast and not have to look and smell presentable in 15 minutes it takes some pressure off and can let you enjoy the sweating.

Instead of interpreting sweating as something dreadful that needs to be cleaned up, shift your thinking to recognize that sweating is a signal that you are working hard, your pores are cleansing, you are releasing heat, and you are doing something good for yourself. Go back to your mindset; accept that sweating is part of caring for your body and shift your perspective about it, looking for the positives.

"I hate to exercise" is often said when we don't know what to do, don't know how to do it or feel embarrassed about how we do it. How did you enjoy moving as a kid? Did you like tag, basketball, gymnastics, swim team? Find an "adult" version that mimics what you enjoyed years ago. If you liked the stop and go of tag you might like boot camp or circuit training. If you loved competition as a kid you might still prefer that. If you loved hula hooping back in the day keep on hula hooping or consider belly dancing now.

Decide what specifically you do and don't like about exercise. Is the idea of being in a gym intimidating? Would you prefer being inside or outside? Would you rather work out alone, with friends or with a group of strangers? Would you prefer moving in water? Do you prefer your exercise time to be loud or quiet and calm? Decide specifically what outcomes you want from exercise and develop a way to achieve those goals.

How to exercise:

The best way to exercise is to do something you enjoy. Do you prefer exercising:

- alone, with a friend or with a group?
- on land or water?
- indoors or outdoors?
- with rhythmic, repetitive movements or freeform movements?
- by competing with a team, competing against yourself or no competition?
- with a trainer or on your own?
- in the morning, afternoon or evening?

Do you need to buy a membership or classes for accountability?

"I hate gyms" is an easy one…don't go. You can create varied and effective exercise routines at home or outdoors. Less gym-ish but still with others are running groups, recreation center exercise classes and sports leagues.

cross training

Exercise can be a fantastic way to reduce stress, but exercise can also be a form of stress for your body. Vigorous and lengthy exercise can at times be too much. Listen to your body and give it a break when it needs it. This can be in the form of a lighter, shorter, easier workout, cross training or skipping a workout to let your body rest.

Cross training is when you alternate between two or more types of exercise that primarily use different muscles: walking and swimming, dancing and yoga, running and rowing, tennis and cycling. You are still exercising but using different muscle groups. Cross training can prevent repetitive use injury, boredom, and can give you a more balanced workout. Having an alternate type of workout can be handy when weather prevents one activity. For example, when it rains for three days and you don't want to walk in the rain you can take a yoga class instead.

create the habit of exercising

Often the hardest part about exercising is just starting. Thinking about it is often worse than doing it. See if you can commit to even just a few minutes each day. It is easier to create the habit of exercising if you have an established time for it daily, even if it is of short duration. Assigning 15 minutes each day six days a week is mentally and physically easier to live with down the road than starting with two 45-minute sessions. As you increase your exercise time it is easier to add on 10 minutes to your existing 15 minutes than it is to carve out two more days for exercise.

By doing it daily you are holding the mental image of you as an exerciser.

plan B

Until frequent exercise becomes a habit and you almost always make time for it you should have a "plan B" for when your initial exercise plans get derailed. Like when your 7 PM walk outside gets cancelled due to a thunderstorm, or you miss a 6 PM spinning class because of traffic, or you hit your snooze button too many times to fit in a swim before work. Without the existence of an alternate plan we might easily give up exercising that day. Knowing in advance what you will do instead eliminates having to think of what to do instead and potentially talk yourself out of doing it.

Plan B is what you do when your original plan falls through. If you don't have time to swim before work could you plan to walk the neighborhood as a backup? When weather cancels outdoor plans could you use a DVD at home?

Think back about what caused you to miss your last few exercise sessions and address the underlying problem. Maybe you don't like exercising alone, or you don't like the type of exercise you are doing. Maybe you don't have the energy after work, or evenings are your most hectic part of the day and you should avoid exercising then.

when to exercise

The best time to exercise is when you will actually do it. Early morning exercise has the benefits of it being done and can't get bumped, it can boost your mood and energy for the day, that time of day has fewer demands, and some people have more energy in the morning. As this time does not appeal to everyone (physically, mentally, or schedule-wise) finding your best time is crucial. When do you have the most energy, control of your schedule and the most potential to follow through with exercising?

how much

Thirty minutes of exercise three times a week is simply not enough. We should be moving daily. And if you are trying to reshape your body you will need to devote more time and intensity than someone looking to maintain what they already achieved. Twenty minutes of intense, devoted exercise is better than forty minutes of half-hearted movement. How long you exercise is determined by what you are trying to accomplish, how you sleep, your stress, and your eating. Be honest about whether your efforts are moving you toward your goals.

There is no magic number or formula for figuring out how much you need to exercise. We are all different and there are many variables. Basically we should be moving throughout each day and exercising daily. If we are trying to lose weight we should move more than someone maintaining weight loss. If you eat a lot you probably need to move a lot. If you move very little you should probably eat less.

• • • •

Exercise enhances your sleep, reduces your stress, boosts your mood and happiness, can improve your eating, and strengthen your willpower. It can be woven into your day in 5-minute increments or done in a continuous stretch. There are so many ways to exercise we should all be able to find two that we can do.

8

happiness

Happiness is a key to living well and has been linked to longevity and a better quality of life. Happy people are more fun to be around. Happiness can draw people to you, thereby letting you enlarge and deepen your social connections. Healthy friendships and relationships play a role in decreasing your stress and increasing your sense of connectedness.

Being happy changes your thoughts and emotions, which ultimately changes your behaviors. Remember, your thoughts drive your behaviors. When you are happy you have more positive thoughts, which results in you making different choices and taking different actions than you might if you are not feeling happy.

defining happiness

Happiness is hard to define. We want it, we can feel it, we recognize it, but just how do we define it? A discussion of happiness touches on the topics of joy, optimism, positivity, resilience, contentment, pleasure, and enjoyment.

We may inaccurately assume that happiness is over the top ecstasy, and that it is normal to live in a constant state of being thrilled and in uncontrolled bliss as portrayed in the media. Happiness is not caused or defined by winning the lottery, fitting in your skinny jeans or buying your dream house. It is much more of an internal job.

Happiness is also not avoiding or eliminating negative feelings. We need to feel all of our feelings. We need to feel all of our emotions to identify them, process them and move on. Dwelling on the negatives is a choice, and so is allowing for more happiness.

gratitude, enjoyment and anticipation: past, present and future

I see happiness as a mix of gratitude, enjoyment and anticipation; it has components from the past, present and future.

gratitude

Gratitude is making the time to note and appreciate things that have already happened. It can be things that made you feel happy, connected, or comfortable, are beautiful, or bring a smile to your face. Don't overlook the little things that make the moment: the sound of children's laughter, someone holding the door for you, enjoying a Popsicle after mowing the grass, a beautiful sunset, a breeze on a warm day, a ray of sunshine on a cold day, or the coziness of your bed.

There is no right or wrong way to practice gratitude. Many people like to start or end their day by thinking about things for which they are grateful. Some people like to write them in a journal, others discuss them with family and still others just review them in their head. Many people like to note a specific number of items. Some people may choose to do a gratitude challenge: come up with way more items than you usually do (if you usually identify 3-5 things, then list 30 or 50). This can force you to think outside your gratitude box.

I like to weave gratitude throughout my day. Periodically I will stop and notice things I am grateful for since the last time I stopped to notice. What could be your reminder to practice gratitude?

When you take a moment to appreciate something don't just note it and quickly move on; stay with it for an extra few seconds to really feel the gratitude. What emotion does that thing bring to you? Staying connected to it even just for a few seconds beyond noticing it can deepen your gratitude and shift it from just a mental exercise to a physical one as well.

The more you stop to notice things you are grateful for, the more things you will notice that make you grateful. It creates a beautiful upward spiral.

enjoyment

Enjoyment is experiencing pleasure in the present moment. We need to occasionally be in the moment or we miss the right now and the opportunity to enjoy things. We rush through life spending most of our time thinking about things from the past or things that might happen in the future but not what is happening right now. When our mind is in the past or future it can't be in the present.

Mindfulness puts you in the present. Whether you are enjoying a meal, a massage, or a gathering of family, slow down and experience it with multiple senses: what you see, smell, taste, hear and touch. Notice also the emotions and feelings it creates. Mindfulness helps boost your enjoyment in the moment.

anticipation

Anticipation is thinking with delight about something that has not happened yet. As children we anticipated so many things. We thought about holidays and birthdays for weeks or months, planning and re-planning what we might like to receive or do. As we got older it became "childish" to spend much time anticipating things. But it's fun to anticipate a date, party, vacation, dream job. Anticipation is not wishing away the present but relishing in the excitement of the future.

Another way to view happiness is to find the balance between having what you want and wanting what you have. If you think about it, this one phrase incorporates the present, past and future. You must be in the moment to notice what you have, you are in the future to identify what you want, and visit the past to want what you have.

boosting happiness

We are each born with a happiness set point. For some people happiness is more elusive but research shows that our set point can be nudged upwards. We can consciously work on becoming happier.

Boosting your happiness is a skill, and you can become happier with practice. Make a conscious effort to notice and think about the good things in life. Once they are in your mind you are more likely to notice even more good things. Live slowly enough that you can enjoy things in the moment.

• • • •

So my secret recipe for happiness is to enjoy the moment, delight in the future and savor things from the past. Happiness boosts your health and wellness and relaxation techniques can boost your happiness. You have more energy, less stress, better sleep and a better quality of life.

21 things you can do to boost your happiness:
1. Practice gratitude.
2. Learn to forgive (let go of grudges).
3. Collect experiences, not stuff.
4. Visualize your best positive future.
5. Live your values.
6. Look for the good.

7. Look for the humor.

8. Look for solutions.

9. Acknowledge that you have the power to change.

10. Think "we" not "me."

11. Each day recommit to being positive.

12. Choose to let your happiness out.

13. Focus on the big picture.

14. Change your perspective from woe to wow.

15. Try something new.

16. Make a decision then move on (stop evaluating whether you made the right decision).

17. Identify 3 strengths, traits or characteristics of which you are proud, then consciously use each strength this week.

18. Focus on relationships.

19. Learn to lessen your stress.

20. Practice random acts of kindness.

21. Be around happy, positive people.

9

motivation

Motivation helps us make healthy changes in eating, exercising, managing stress, boosting happiness, getting better sleep and tweaking our thoughts. It supports all aspects of our wellness.

We need a plan for keeping our new, healthy behaviors in motion until they become habits. Motivation is what keeps us going while we have to consciously think about doing things. It keeps our sleep, eating, stress management, gratitude, and exercising on track. Once something becomes a habit we do not need to spend time thinking about doing it and it no longer requires a lot of mental energy.

Making lifestyle changes is a gradual process. You keep working on each change: maintaining your successes, repeating the behaviors until they become habits and pushing yourself forward with new goals. Once a behavior becomes a habit you do not need the same level of attention and focus to maintain it, it becomes automatic. Maintaining motivation takes effort and awareness. There will be periods where it seems easy and periods when it seems difficult.

You can't maintain changes unless your thoughts and beliefs support the changes. Just going through the motions is not sustainable. Take time to check in with your thoughts, values and beliefs. Sometimes your thoughts need a tune-up to stay in alignment with your goals and vision.

willpower

Staying motivated is easier when we see positive results and our willpower feels strong. Willpower is like a muscle; it can be both strengthened and exhausted. We need to stay aware of what drains our willpower (stress, decisions, annoyances, fatigue, hunger, boredom, overwhelm) and what we can do to replenish our willpower (relax, sleep, eat, exercise, and positive thinking).

achieving and maintaining

Achieving a goal and maintaining it are different skill sets. In the achieving mode your enthusiasm starts out high, the idea is fresh, people support your new endeavor, you have not yet had setbacks and you are at peak motivation. You are more focused on putting one foot in front of the other. Maintaining what you achieved is a different story. You are trying to weave the new behavior into your lifestyle and as you get more accustomed to the behavior you can feel far from it feeling effortless. People no longer notice all of your accomplishments, you feel more isolated and like you are doing the same motion over and over. In maintenance you need to be your primary cheerleader and encourager.

motivation curve

Motivation and enthusiasm follow a U-shaped curve. You start out very excited and confident. Then comes a period where it seems like hard work, you aren't seeing progress and you feel like giving up. If you keep working toward your goal your energy and results start picking back up and your motivation and excitement move upward again. Think of a long car trip that you have made several times. You are excited to go and have lots of energy in the beginning. You plan and pack and people wish you a fun and safe trip and wave goodbye. You are driving and driving, and no one at rest stops congratulates you on the progress you have made. You are so far from your starting point and end point that you can't see either one. Your motivation slumps. Then the trip becomes drudgery; the scenery is boring, the driving is tedious, you only want to be at your destination. You need to get back in the car and keep driving knowing that your destination is out there and has to be getting closer with each mile. As you reach the last leg of the trip and are close to your destination your enthusiasm picks up again. You are close enough to see and feel the endpoint and the drive becomes enjoyable again. The same is true when making lifestyle changes.

avoid comparisons

Avoid comparing yourself to others. We all have something we are working on and your "thing" may not be the same as another person's; your circumstances may be wildly different. We all need different forms and amounts of exercise, food, and sleep. Our stress levels and happiness vary. We are all similar yet unique. You are not on the same exact journey as anyone else; you might want to reach the same destination but your journey will look different. And that's a beautiful thing!

seeing the forest and the trees

- Always know where you are going.

- Step back and admire all that you have accomplished so far but keep an eye to the future.

- Create the ability to see both the forest and the trees. The forest is the big picture that keeps you moving forward. The trees are the small details, the individual baby steps. You need to see them long enough to step past them but not long enough to get lost and lose sight of the final destination.

- Drive looking forward, occasionally checking the rear view mirror.

- Know why you are making the changes.

- Envision the future; see it, feel it, make it seem real right now.

- Remind yourself you can do this.

- Keep taking action.

- Check your beliefs.

- Focus on positive thoughts, reframe negativity.

- Break your goals into small action steps.

- Keep taking baby steps.

- Look for progress, drop the desire for perfection.

- Maximize your willpower. Plan ahead for the times of day, week, month that you know are more difficult. Accept that willpower waxes and wanes and plan for it.

- Create and use support systems.

- Nourish your body, mind and soul.

- Recommit each day (or even each hour or minute) to staying the course.

- You have choices to make, and the power to choose well!

• • • •

Your motivation will sustain you through the changes involved in creating a lifestyle of wellness. Your sleep, stress, eating, exercise, happiness and mindset all play a role in your health and wellness. They are all intertwined and all support each other. Keep moving forward. Your thoughts drive your behaviors and taking action boosts your confidence.

Making a journey analogy for staying motivated:

- decide where you are going and how you will know when you get there
- keep your map out
- drive looking forward, occasionally checking the rearview mirror
- refuel before running out of gas
- ask for directions (support) when you need them
- plan for detours
- notice your progress, there is no perfect route
- don't get discouraged when the last 50 miles looked monotonous
- enjoy the scenery along the way, stop and visit towns, notice the details
- keep driving
- its ok to change your destination
- enjoy the ride

10

integrated again

The foot bone is connected to the leg bone and the leg bone is connected to the hip bone...Creating wellness is a process of acknowledging and maximizing the interconnectedness of our body, mind and spirit. We are all capable of making monumental changes, one small step at a time.

Our thoughts, beliefs, and mindset both drive and stabilize our ability to move forward. Our mind affects our body and our behaviors. How we manage our time creates the space in which we exercise, eat well, manage our stress, sleep, and make time for happiness. And motivation keeps us moving forward.

Stress affects our health. When our stress is managed well we:

- make better food choices

- are more patient and creative

- have a stronger immune system

- have a more efficient metabolism

- have more energy

- are more likely to exercise

- have a better mood and mindset

- sleep better

Adequate sleep:

- boosts our energy

- improves our mood

- reduces our stress

- makes us more likely to make better food choices

- improves our odds of exercising

Better eating:

- gives us more energy

- reduces stress

- improves our chances of exercising

- helps us sleep better
- improves our mood

Exercising:

- reduces stress
- enhances sleep
- boosts our mood
- can improve our food choices
- give us more energy

Happiness:

- feels great
- can enhance good food choices
- improves sleep
- reduces stress
- makes us more likely to exercise

Wellness also includes keeping an eye on your thoughts, treating yourself with compassion, and looking for progress and positives. Change starts with awareness and moves forward with action. What's your next step?

Enjoy your journey!

your next step

I thank you for reading this book and am honored to be part of your wellness journey.

Your wellness journey includes an amalgam of integrated pieces: your mindset, stress management, time management, eating, sleep, exercise, happiness, and motivation. Each component affects and is affected by the other components. Together they make a whole you.

Positive changes in any section can cause positive changes elsewhere in your wellness, creating that beautiful continuous spiral. The journey really can be quite simple; not necessarily easy, but simple. You absolutely can do this. Keep taking action.

If you enjoyed *Wellness Made Simple,* share it with your friends and please visit my website: www.YouBloomWellness.com for information on coaching, a relaxation CD, and upcoming books and events.

You can also sign up for my complimentary e-zine *Ideas for Living Well,* which comes out every other week with a short article and tips on managing stress, better eating, exercise, happiness, and improving your wellness.

Visit my website to download a free guided imagery re-laxation exercise: www.YouBloomWellness.com.

If you would like more support on your path to wellness consider joining a group coaching program or talking to me about 1:1 coaching (both done by phone so you can conveniently do it from your home no matter where that is!).

If you want to hear this information live, invite me to speak to your organization. Check the corporate wellness page on my website for topics or contact me to discuss a specific idea.

Take your next step; put the information into action!

Laura

about laura

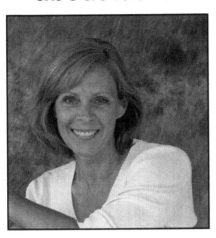

Laura is an RN, speaker, and certified wellness coach living in Pittsburgh, PA with her children, bunnies and a leopard gecko. She loves rabbits, dark chocolate, gardening, and lava lamps. Leaving patient care allowed her to focus on helping people take a proactive role in their wellness. Through coaching and speaking she helps people feeling flabby, crabby and overwhelmed feel fit, energetic and enthusiastic.

For more information please visit www.YouBloomWellness.com.

60570491R00086

Made in the USA
Charleston, SC
04 September 2016